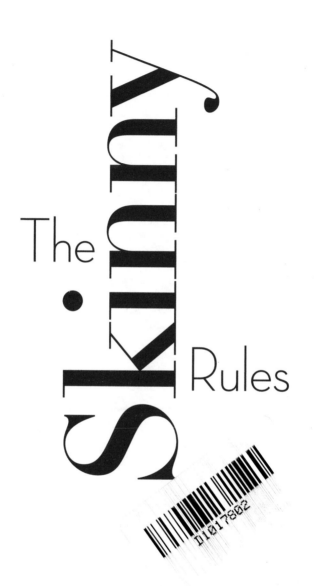

The Skinny Rules

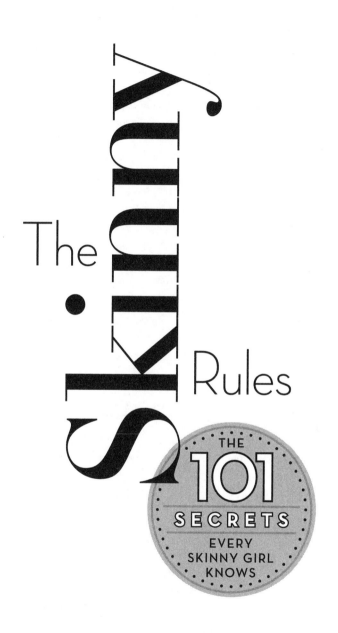

The Skinny Rules

THE 101 SECRETS EVERY SKINNY GIRL KNOWS

MOLLY MORGAN, RD, CDN

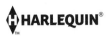

The Skinny Rules

ISBN: 978-0-373-89228-0

© 2011 by Molly Morgan, RD, CDN

The ideas, procedures and suggestions contained in this book are not intended as a substitute for consulting with your physician. All matters regarding your health require medical supervision.

Library of Congress Cataloging-in-Publication Data
Morgan, Molly.
The skinny rules : the 101 secrets every skinny girl knows/ Molly Morgan.
     p. cm.
Includes bibliographical references and index.
ISBN 978-0-373-89228-0 (pbk.)
1. Reducing diets—Juvenile literature. 2. Reducing exercises—Juvenile literature. 3. Girls—Health and hygiene—Juvenile literature. I. Title.

RM222.2.M5687 2011
613.2'5—dc22

                    2010024187

www.eHarlequin.com

Printed in U.S.A.

To my husband and our two little men.

Contents

CONTENTS

4 | Skinny Cooking 101

5   Skinny Parties and Travel 133

6   Skinny Eating Out 161

Acknowledgments

First and foremost, I have to thank my husband, who put up with my long hours at the computer typing away to get this book written, and our little guys, who were as understanding as a baby and toddler can be about their mommy needing to work.

This book became a reality thanks to Holly Schmidt: I can't thank her enough for her time and dedication bringing this project to life and to Sarah Pelz, my editor from Harlequin who helped to guide the writing and corrected every page of this book.

Last but not least is a thank-you to the numerous outstanding experts who provided tips and content for this book, who are all listed in Appendix A. Their time and effort in providing expertise is much appreciated.

Introduction

I was writing this book at the most ironic point in my life. To make a long story short, I signed the publishing contract when our second son was only three weeks old, at a time when most women feel the furthest thing from "Skinny." Which brings me to my first point—what does it mean to be Skinny? Society has defined *Skinny* as what size clothes you wear and how you look in them. The medical community defines *Skinny* by your body mass index (BMI)—the ratio of your height to your weight. And the dictionary defines *Skinny* as: *being thin.*

Yet, as a nutrition expert, I have my own definition of *Skinny.* I believe that *Skinny* is actually defined by the lifestyle you lead and not by the size clothes you wear. Let's say your BMI is in a "healthy range" and you appear visibly thin—does this mean you are healthy? I say maybe. If you are eating well, exercising and taking care of your body then, yes, this is living a *healthy* Skinny life. If you are filling your body with garbage foods, smoking, and are inactive then, no, even if you appear Skinny, you aren't living a Skinny life! My goal is to challenge you to think of Skinny in a new way—think of it as living a healthy and active life, rather than defining *Skinny* simply by the size clothes you wear.

Now take a moment and ask yourself who are you trying to be "Skinny" for? Here is a piece of advice that I love. It comes from Alison Sweeney, host of *The Biggest Loser,* who told www.fitnessmagazine.com, "Do it for yourself! If you're trying to lose weight for your husband or mother, it won't work." If you are trying to change your lifestyle for someone else, you aren't going to have the true motivation you need to change. Challenge yourself to change your mind-set and focus on getting Skinny for you—not someone else!

As a registered dietitian, people often ask me what I think about the "obesity epidemic"—why the rates of obesity and overweight individuals are soaring worldwide, and especially in the United States. I don't think there is just one factor; there are lots and lots of factors. As my husband says, "You don't catch fat!" What he means is that it isn't as if one morning you wake up 50 pounds heavier than the day before. Gaining weight happens over time and losing weight takes time. There aren't any magic pills or powders or potions that will do the work for you; instead, there are Skinny rules you can follow to adjust your lifestyle to take the weight off.

Did you like those "choose your own adventure" books as a child? I certainly did! As I was writing this book, it struck me that losing weight and becoming a healthier version of you is kind of like choosing your own adventure! You can even think of this book as your choose-your-own food, nutrition, cooking, fitness and fashion rule book, filled with tips, tricks and secrets to get you on a path to a healthier and Skinnier you! Let the adventure begin!

One

Surprising Skinny Rules

Believe You
Can Be Skinny

The first Skinny rule is that you must believe you can be Skinny. This is one rule that all Skinny girls follow—they don't question whether or not it's possible to be thin and stay that way. They just do it.

You must know that losing weight *is possible!* Every day, we're bombarded with depressing statistics and numbers about how many people are overweight, but what we really need to be hearing is less about the saddening stats and more about what you can actually do to adopt a healthy lifestyle! Throughout this book you will be reading rules that can and will help you meet your goals in a healthful way.

This rule was inspired by Cynthia Sass, MPH, MA, RD, CSSD, a New York City–based registered dietitian and the bestselling co-author of *Flat Belly Diet!* As she explains, "So often we hear that diets and exercise don't work, but I've worked with hundreds of people over the years who have lost weight healthfully and kept it off." Her motivating tip is this: "Don't give up—it's about finding what works for you and choices that make you feel good both physically and emotionally that you can stick with."

Skinny Rule #1 is all about your frame of mind. You have to start talking positively to yourself and psyching yourself up that you can do this! This component is crucial. Because even after you read this book, you will have lots of ways—101 ways—to shape up your lifestyle and become a thinner version of you, but *you* are the one who has to do the work. So before you read on, start telling yourself that it's possible! Believe you can be Skinny. Whenever you feel that it isn't possible, jump right back to this page and read it again! This one simple rule can make all the difference for you.

As a reminder, jot down, "It's possible" or "I believe" on a sticky note and post it on your desk, your bathroom mirror or, better yet, on your refrigerator, reminding yourself throughout the day that it *is* possible to drop pounds healthfully and keep them off. You won't find any crazy powders, pills or promises in this book, but you will find all the to-the-point tips, tricks and rules to guide you on the path to a healthier, Skinnier version of you. So now that you know you can do it, let's get started! ⓢ

| SKINNY RULE 2 | Hit the Pillow |

This is one of the most surprising Skinny rules, as it has nothing to do with what you eat or how much you exercise, but believe it or not, sleep is just as important! Skinny girls think of sleep as a necessity, not a luxury, and they never miss out on any precious ZZZs. That's because sleep is a Skinny essential—it plays a crucial role in controlling your appetite.

Getting less than the recommended seven to nine hours of sleep per night increases your odds of being overweight and having a higher body fat percentage. It even puts you at risk for type 2 diabetes. Why? Research shows that sleep affects the levels of leptin and ghrelin in the body, two hormones that control and stimulate hunger.

Leptin is a Skinny secret weapon because one of the key roles it plays is to tell your brain: *Hey! Stop eating, I'm full!* When you sleep, your levels of leptin increase, letting your body know that it has plenty of energy and there's no need to trigger the feeling of hunger. Scientists are still trying to understand more precisely how this hormone works.

So while science tries to further explain it, what is known is that when you aren't getting enough sleep, your body winds up with lower levels of this Skinny, appetite-controlling hormone, which leaves you feeling hungry even when you really don't need food!

While more leptin means you feel less hungry, the opposite is true of ghrelin. Ghrelin tells your brain when you need to eat and while you sleep, levels of ghrelin decrease because sleep requires less energy than what is needed when you are awake. When you aren't getting enough sleep, you actually wind up having more of the appetite-stimulating hormone in your system, which makes your body believe it is hungry.

By getting a full night's rest, you help your body recharge leptin levels and decrease ghrelin levels to keep your appetite in check all day long.

The good news is that there are plenty of things you can do to help make sure you are getting enough sleep. Take a look at your schedule and adjust it to allow for more time to sleep. Have dinner at least two to three hours before bed to give your body enough time to digest the food.

If you are going to have a night snack, have it about one hour before bedtime and keep it light, simple and small. A combination of carbohydrates and protein is the perfect sleep-friendly combination because the carbohydrates provide the amino acid tryptophan that naturally relaxes the brain and has a calming effect. Try these great sleep-inducing snack ideas: a few whole-grain crackers and light cheese, a bowl of whole-grain cereal with milk or a glass of warm milk.

If you're still having trouble, check out these sleep tips from the National Sleep Foundation:

- Have a bedtime routine that is relaxing; try listening to soothing music and being calm an hour or so before you want to be asleep.
- Make sure your sleeping environment is comfortable, dark and cool.

- Plan your exercise to end at least a few hours before bedtime.
- Close to bedtime, give up smoking and avoid caffeine. ⓢⓡ

SKINNY RULE 3

Skip the Sauce

Here's the deal and it's something that Skinny girls swear by: Next time you sit down to eat, think twice before you start dipping your foods in salad dressings or condiments. Why? That side of ketchup may look harmless, but it's packed with tons of carbs! In just three tablespoons of ketchup there are almost as many carbohydrates as in a slice of bread and about 45 calories. You may think, what's the big deal with having an extra 45 calories? Well, having just an extra 45 calories a day over the course of a year equals 16,425 calories or over 4½ pounds' worth of calories—that's practically a whole dress size, thanks to ketchup!

Other sauces are even worse offenders. In just two little tablespoons of ranch dressing, about the size of a shot glass, there are about 148 calories. Once you start dipping your otherwise-healthy fresh broccoli in dressing, you're piling up unnecessary calories and extra unwanted fat, to the tune of about 16 grams of fat per two tablespoons. Do this even just twice a week and over the course of the year it will pile up to equal about 15,392 calories or another four pounds' worth of calories!

Mayonnaise is another dressing that can add calories in a hurry, weighing in at about 100 calories for just one tablespoon. Having mayonnaise on a sandwich only one time a week over the course of a year would equal 5,200 calories or a pound and a half's worth of calories!

Take a look again at the three examples listed on the previous page. Skipping the mayo, salad dressing and ketchup could save about 10 pounds' worth of calories over a year! So follow the Skinny rule: Skip the sauce and save the calories! 🆂🆁

<table>
<tr><td>SKINNY
RULE
4</td><td># Record It</td></tr>
</table>

T his is one of my favorite Skinny rules: Recording your progress will help you stay on track and help you see how far you've really come. Plus, it can help you identify what may be working for or against getting you to meet your Skinny goals. And there are plenty of different ways to record your Skinny life.

One of my favorite success stories is from a woman I coached to help lose those last five pounds and achieve her goal weight. She kept what we called, a "little black book," which was a cute cloth-covered notebook where she jotted down her daily weight checks, food intake and thoughts and feelings about her progress. The power of this little black book came around the second year of its use because we could look back and see how far she had come and celebrate her Skinny successes!

Or if you're into taking pictures, maybe you can do what supermodel Heidi Klum does. As she shared with www.nowloss.com, her Skinny secret to losing 30 pounds in the first six months after giving birth was to take photographs of herself every week in the nude to keep track of the way her body was changing. Why did this work? It motivated her to keep making healthy choices and visually monitor the progress that she was making.

Or you could record your progress on a number of websites. My husband swears by the website www.mapmyride.com; it has helped him take off more than 30 pounds. This site helps you record your daily exercise and what's especially cool is that once you log in your workouts, it calculates how many calories you burned. Then you can look at how many calories you burned in a week or a month. This can be a really effective way to evaluate and track your fitness progress.

If that's not your thing, you can make a note in your day planner that simply says "exercise" or "no exercise." Just the basic routine of making yourself write down whether or not you exercised may be just enough to make you get up earlier or squeeze in that workout!

Perhaps even better yet, work with a registered dietitian (RD) to record how you are doing with your eating and exercise regimen. Taking the time for a quick check-in with an RD once a week may be what you need to keep recording your progress, moving forward and living a Skinny life. In fact, many RDs will even do web- or phone-based consultations so you don't have to take the time out of your schedule to go to the RD's office.

The bottom line is that what works for you may be different than what will work for someone else. There isn't a right or wrong way to record your Skinny progress—just doing it is the key! 𝕊ℝ

| SKINNY RULE 5 | Get on the Scale |

In my estimation, getting on the scale is one of the single most important steps that Skinny girls do. Let me explain.

If you avoid the scale like the plague (no judgment—you're not alone!) and then weigh in at your annual checkup only to realize you have gained 10 pounds, it's going to be difficult to shed those new pounds. But if you had checked your weight routinely (at least every few days), you would have noticed the gradual increase in the numbers on the scale and could have done something about it before they added up!

One great example of this is the National Weight Control Registry, an inspiring group of over 5,000 people who are tracked because they've lost 30 pounds or more and kept it off. And a significant 75 percent report that they check their weight at least once a week.

In Skinny Rule #4 on page 6, I introduced a woman who recorded her progress in a little black book. Part of her record included her daily weight checks and her thoughts and feelings about them. Sometimes those thoughts were happy and other times those thoughts were four-letter words, but monitoring those ups and downs is all part of the Skinny process. Writing down her weight on an almost daily basis also helped her understand what her typical weight fluctuations are. Everyone's weight will fluctuate—a woman's weight by about three pounds per day and a man's weight by about five pounds per day. Keeping this little black book helped her to realize, for example, that after eating out at restaurants her weight typically took a three-pound leap, but within a few days those pounds were gone. This is a crucial point to understand, so that you don't panic at every fluctuation. Those pounds are not what I like to call "sticky" pounds; rather, they are just a natural fluctuation in your weight.

Some may argue that checking your weight daily can lead to an obsession about weight, but I beg to differ. I believe that checking your weight daily can help you better understand and be more at peace with your weight and how it changes. It also allows you to quickly pick up on unwanted weight gain. (If you do find that you're obsessing over your weight, this could be a sign of a more serious problem and I would recommend talking with your doctor.)

Now with all this talk about weight, how do you figure out how much you should weigh? The best place to start is the Body Mass Index (BMI) chart. Although it certainly has its limitations, it is a starting point to determine what is a healthy weight range for your height. Check out the link to this Skinny tool in Appendix B (the National Institutes of Health, Body Mass Index Chart).

Yet keep in mind that weight is a tricky thing and depends on many factors. You can't always go by the scale or guidelines alone. For example, if some of the professional athletes I work with relied on the BMI chart, they would think that they need to lose weight. In fact, they are at the top of their sport and in excellent shape; their weight is simply higher than the average person's because of increased muscle mass. Does this person truly need to lose weight? No! And remember, "Skinny" is more than just a number on the scale or the pants size you wear: If you're at a healthy weight for your height but not eating healthy and exercising, then you're not living the true Skinny life! 🆂🆁

SKINNY RULE 6

Skip the Soft Drinks—*Even Diet*

Everyone knows that regular soft drinks are loaded with empty calories, but it turns out that diet soda isn't diet-friendly, either! The San Antonio Heart Study, a twenty-five-year-long study conducted at the University of Texas Health Science Center at San Antonio, found that the more diet soda a person drinks, the greater chance that she will become overweight. "On average, for each diet soft drink our participants drank per day, they were 65 percent more likely to become overweight during the next seven to eight years, and 41 percent more likely to become obese," said Sharon Fowler, MPH, faculty associate in the division of clinical epidemiology in the Health Science Center's Department of Medicine.

Perhaps even more interesting is that the researchers found a dose-related response. Those who guzzled down the most diet soft drinks actually had the highest frequency of weight gain. While unsure of the exact cause of the weight gain, Fowler and her colleagues speculate that it may be related, in part, to the participants' cutback in or lack of nutrient-rich drinks like milk, and the lack of plain old water. Another possibility is that participants who drank diet soft drinks did so because they were trying to stop weight gain or lose weight.

In addition, could there be a relationship between the intensely sweet flavor of the drinks and increased food intake? One theory of mine is that the heightened sweetness of diet drinks actually makes us crave more sweets and results in our eating more sweet foods, like candy, which tend to provide empty calories. This theory stems from my own personal experience with virtually eliminating diet sodas from my eating routine. Now whenever I do have a rare diet soda, it tastes intensely sweet. But when I had them on a regular basis that supersweet taste seemed like the norm.

While the jury is still out on the exact reason diet drinks are linked to obesity, use the correlation as motivation to cut down on the amount of diet beverages you drink. When I asked celebrity personal trainer Michael George for the Skinny rules that he personally lives by, one of his rules was drinking "water, water, and more water!" Remember, plain water is the original calorie-free beverage—it's nothing but good for you. Instead of turning to sugar or sugar substitute–sweetened beverages, have a glass of water—you can even perk it up with a few lemon, lime or cucumber slices! ⓢ

SKINNY
RULE
7

Be a Work in Progress

An important component of living a Skinny life is to be a work in progress. As Robyn Priebe, RD, CDN, the director of nutrition at Green Mountain at Fox Run Spa, explains, "living a healthy lifestyle is a process that occurs over time."

Priebe wants all her clients to be a work in progress: She advises them to do periodic self-assessments to identify any improvements they can make in their current eating habits. This process is critical because it ensures that you don't get stuck in a rut with one particular way of eating. Additionally, continuous self-assessment can help to quickly identify problem areas and what you need to change. Most important, it allows you to make small, manageable changes over time, rather than overhauling your diet in one fell swoop.

For example, make it part of your routine to ask yourself every Friday: Have I been drinking enough water throughout the week? Have I been eating enough fruit? Have I been eating enough vegetables? Have I been keeping my portions in check at dinner and planning my meals? If you answer no to any of these questions, this self-assessment allows you to quickly pick up on a potential problem area that needs improvement in your diet before it becomes a routine or bad habit.

Self-assessments are also an opportunity to pinpoint any issues you may have with emotional eating. When you overate last week or craved sugary foods, was it correlated with a stressful or hectic week at work? Identifying that you are an emotional eater is half the battle. Once you recognize these emotional triggers, you can prepare in advance to sidestep emotional eating by dealing with your emotions in ways other than eating. Instead of eating to cope with stress, take the Skinny approach and take a walk, go for a run, clean your house or call a friend. While some of those activities burn more calories than others, they are all calorie savers if they keep you from eating to deal with your feelings.

Another key to being a work in progress is to cut yourself some slack—after all, food is part of our everyday life and life is continuously changing and presenting new challenges. Giving yourself this permission is a perfect way to keep upbeat and stay realistic about reaching your Skinny goals. Otherwise, you could go crazy in the process! 🆂🆁

SKINNY RULE 8	Get in the Driver's Seat

This could arguably be the most important Skinny rule of them all, and it certainly pertains to more than just weight and health: Skinny girls get in the driver's seat; they take charge and full responsibility for their life, weight and health! In other words, they hold themselves accountable. (For more on accountability, see Skinny Rule #9.)

So often I hear new patients tell me that they're stuck in a vicious cycle of jumping from diet to diet, or continually going back to a diet that failed them in the past. The truth is, it isn't the diets that have failed—it's that they aren't making consistent changes. And who can blame them? Dieting is no way to live at all! Skinny people take charge of their health and diet and create a plan that works for them—and what works for one person will not necessarily work for the next. Actually, I think Albert Einstein said it best: "The definition of insanity is doing the same thing over and over again and expecting different results." Get in the driver's seat and figure out a plan that works for you.

As part of Skinny Rule #8, you need to know yourself well. For example, let's say you read an article that says that people who are vegetarians tend to weigh less, but you hate vegetables. Is becoming a vegetarian really a good solution for you to get healthy and lose weight? I would say no. As the driver, you need to know what will work for you and be realistic about it. That's the only way you'll be able to steer yourself in the right direction.

I will use myself as an example. While going to a gym to exercise works great for some people, for me it is a recipe for a lot of wasted money. Why? I don't like working out in a gym. Instead, I have hand weights, sneakers, a bike, skis, exercise DVDs, yoga mats and the like at home, which allow me to enjoy all sorts of different types of exercise and work exercise into my routine much more easily than if I have to go to a gym to work out.

As the driver, you get to determine what will work best for you, making it much more likely that you'll arrive at destination Skinny. ®

| SKINNY RULE 9 | Call on a Co-Pilot |

Now that you're in the driver's seat and have taken responsibility for your diet, it's time to invite some passengers to join you. To support you on your journey, you need to call on a co-pilot, or maybe even a car full of people to bolster your efforts along the way. This is definitely true when it comes to your health. Of course you need a health care provider, but you also need someone to help hold you accountable for your fitness and eating routines.

If you're having a hard time coming up with a plan, a registered dietitian (RD) is a great "co-pilot" to call on. RDs can create a custom plan to meet your goals. You can find a registered dietitian by going to www.eatright.org and clicking on "Find a Registered Dietitian." Wherever you search, be sure to enlist a registered dietitian and not just a nutritionist, because RDs have formal schooling in nutrition and have to maintain their registration through a series of continuing education requirements every five years.

Now you may need other people in your car to help steer you on the right path. Add family members or friends to your team and call on them for support when you are having a tough time staying motivated to lose weight. You may want to enlist the support of a personal trainer to help fine-tune or establish a fitness routine for you. Make sure that your personal trainer is a CPT, Certified Personal Trainer. There are many different personal training certificate programs, so if you are unsure if someone is qualified, ask what type of training program he went through and you can look up that program to make sure that it is legitimate.

Who else should you add to your car? Some people may need to add a therapist to their car, especially if they are struggling with any sort of emotional eating issues. A social worker or psychologist can help work with you to calm your emotions and address any potential issues that may arise when you are trying to make lifestyle changes.

Stop and think for a moment: Who is going to be in your car? The answer to this question will be different for everyone and may even change for you from time to time. Nonetheless, don't feel ashamed if you need the support of others. Rather, embrace their support; it will surely help you meet your goals. 🆂🆁

SKINNY
RULE
10

Opt for Fast Food over Restaurants

Everyone knows that fast food is bad for you, but could it be that fast food restaurants have been getting a bad rap for no good reason? In many cases, fast food menu options weigh in with fewer calories than their sit-down restaurant counterparts! Amazing, huh?

Research proves this very point. A recent study in the journal *Applied Economic Perspectives and Policy,* comparing calories for sit-down restaurants, fast food restaurants and home-cooked meals, concluded that sit-down restaurants have larger portions and, therefore, more calories than fast food places. Not surprisingly, eating at home proves to be the healthiest option of the three.

Here is a recent real-world example: My husband and I do not eat out a lot and avoid fast food like the plague, so it never occurred to me that fast food might be healthier than restaurant food. But when I looked into the facts and did a little research, the reality took me by surprise. My husband and I were traveling and we sought out a Ruby Tuesday's that was just about 30 minutes ahead on our route and placed an order to go, thinking this would be a healthier option than stopping at a fast food restaurant.

I ordered a turkey burger with a side salad (instead of fries) and my husband opted for the mini burger trio and fries. After we had eaten I looked up the nutrition facts for our menu items. While I knew that what we had just eaten wasn't health food by any stretch of the imagination, I was shocked to find that my turkey burger had a whopping 890 calories and 48 grams of fat and my husband's mini burger meal (including the fries) had 1,215 calories and 60 grams of fat! The worst part about this is that we thought we were making a healthier choice by avoiding fast food.

We could have gone through the drive-thru at any fast food place and picked up a meal with fewer calories. Check out these comparisons:

Food Item	Fast Food Restaurant (Burger King)	Sit-Down Restaurant (Ruby Tuesday)
Classic Cheeseburger	300 calories for 1 burger	999 calories for 1 burger
Grilled Chicken Sandwich	470 calories for 1 sandwich	869 calories for 1 sandwich
French Fries	340 calories for a small order	396 calories for a side order
Grilled Chicken Salad	490 calories for 1 salad	701 calories for 1 salad

The menu item that shocked me the most was the grilled chicken sandwich at the sit-down restaurant—869 calories, yikes!

Knowledge is power: Learn from my mistake and look up the nutrition facts for the menu items that you're interested in ordering before you place your order. This will allow you to adjust your order to reduce calories, which is especially important if you dine out frequently. Most restaurants post nutrition facts on their website or you can request a copy of them at the restaurant. Check out Part Six: Skinny Eating Out for more tips and tricks on eating Skinny when you eat out. ⑤

| SKINNY RULE **11** | Skinny-Size These Fattening Foods |

S kinny girls don't deprive themselves. If they are in the mood for a bagel, pasta or a creamy dip, they go for it. But they indulge the Skinny way. Rather than avoiding the foods you love, try these Skinny secrets to cut calories, without cutting flavor.

SKINNY BAGELS: Nutrition expert and American Dietetic Association spokesperson Keri Gans suggests scooping your bagel. What to do: Take a spoon and scoop out the inside dough of the bagel. Why bother? Well, one bagel is approximately equal to eating four to five slices of bread! By scooping out the inside of a bagel, you will be scooping away calories while still enjoying the delicious taste. After you scoop out a bagel, try filling it with a light spread of creamy cream cheese and fresh berries. It's the perfect Skinny way to enjoy a bagel! If you are really serious about scooping, check out the Lé Scoop bagel scooper (see Appendix B), a Skinny kitchen must-have.

SKINNY OIL: One of my favorite calorie-cutting, Skinny secrets is to use an olive oil mister. Olive oil is a wonderful, heart-healthy fat, but each tablespoon has about 120 calories and 14 grams of fat, which means those calories can pile up quickly. An olive oil mister will allow you to use the heart-healthy oil in your cooking while controlling the amount used and, in turn, cutting calories. When you pour olive oil from the bottle to use for cooking, it is easy to overdo it. And even if you use a measuring spoon to carefully measure the amount of oil that you are adding, you can still use less with the mister! For example, when you are stir-frying, let's say you would typically use one tablespoon (equal to three teaspoons) of olive oil; with an olive oil mister every spray is only one-quarter of a teaspoon, which is only 10 calories. That means you can spray four sprays from your mister and still have only 40 calories, which is a quarter of the number of calories as compared to the tablespoon that you would have used. The bottom line is that you have just saved about 80 calories! Do this every time you cook and the calorie savings will pile up in a hurry. Head to a kitchen store and pick up an olive oil mister or refill a mister from a marinade or salad dressing. For more must-have Skinny cooking tools, see Part Four: Skinny Cooking.

SKINNY DIPS: There is a surefire Skinny rule to cutting calories when making creamy salads and dips. The secret is to replace the mayonnaise with plain, low-fat yogurt. Making this swap will save about 400 calories and 42 grams of fat per cup! This calorie-saving secret will allow you to still enjoy creamy salads and dips without the guilt and the unwanted calories. If you're hesitant to make the change, start by substituting half the high-calorie mayonnaise with plain, low-fat yogurt.

SKINNY PASTA: Pasta—you've always thought of it as the ultimate forbidden food. But now it doesn't have to be. Kristine Schoembs, a cousin of mine who has been enjoying living at a healthy weight since 2004, shares her secret to enjoying pasta the Skinny way! She fills her pasta bowl with baby spinach and then tops it with whole-wheat pasta and sauce. The warm pasta steams the spinach and this way she still enjoys a yummy dish of pasta but eats a lot less because the spinach really makes the bowl look full. Plus the spinach adds a boost of antioxidants, thanks to its deep, dark green color, and the dish also boasts lots of belly-filling fiber! Next time you make pasta for a meal, try Kristine's Skinny solution! ⓢⓡ

SKINNY RULE 12

Walk the Walk

With all the diet information in the media today, we all seem to think we are experts on nutrition. I can't tell you how many times I have heard people say, "I know what to do. I just need to figure out how to do it." This is where Skinny Rule #12 comes in: You have to walk the walk. Rather than just talking about how you heard that getting enough sleep every night helps to control your appetite, you need to figure out how to fit a good night's rest into your life. Or rather than talking about how you should start eating breakfast every day when you hit that energy low around 11:00 a.m. in the office, start eating it. You need to start making Skinny changes in your life and create a plan that will work for you.

This is especially true for moms and dads: You're role models for your children when it comes to food and nutrition. You may not even realize how powerful a role you play. Think about this for a minute. If you are sitting down to a meal and you pour yourself a fizzy, sugary soft drink, yet you make your children consume milk with their dinner, what kind of message are you sending? When you step back and think about it, you are certainly sending your children a mixed message. Skinny people live more by the *Do as I say and as I do* motto rather than *Do as I say, not as I do.*

So how can you start walking the walk? The answer to this question will be different for every person. Maybe you need to start buying more fruit. Maybe you need to scale back on how often you eat out. Perhaps you need to try a new recipe once a week. Even invest some money in kitchen or exercise supplies to make it easier, more convenient and more feasible to meet your goals. And the great thing about walking the walk is that you can think of it as literally taking steps to living a healthier, Skinnier life. ⓢⓡ

SKINNY RULE 13

Give Your Meal a Makeover

Figuring out what to make for dinner can be a challenge, especially when it seems like you have the same meals over and over again. Your taste buds get bored when dinner becomes redundant. Making over your meals is a Skinny rule to get you to enjoy healthier foods while keeping your taste buds happy.

Alternate Your Sides

One simple way to add variety to your meal plan is to switch your side dishes. There's no need to pour on heavy sauces or load your side dishes with butter. Limit side dishes to veggies, fruit or whole grains. These foods will add delicious flavor, a variety of colors and, of course, curb the total calories in your meal. Some of my favorite Skinny side dishes include:

EDAMAME: Buy the shelled variety and simply steam or microwave them for a perfectly delicious, protein-packed side dish.

SWEET POTATOES: Although they get a bad rap for their carbohydrate count, they are loaded with nutrients and belly-filling fiber.

MANGO: Simply cube a fresh mango and serve it with grilled fish, pork chops, even chicken for a flavorful side dish.

WHOLE-GRAIN COUSCOUS: Prepare the couscous according to package instructions and season with garlic powder or your favorite spice blend.

> When you're grilling veggies like carrots or potatoes, cook them in the microwave or on the stovetop for a few minutes to soften them a bit. This will shorten your grilling time.
>
> Skinny Tip

BABY SPINACH: Sautéed with a small amount of extra virgin olive oil and balsamic vinegar.

Use Skinny Cooking Techniques

The Skinniest way to make over a meal and add flavor without piling on calories is by switching your cooking methods. Here are a few Skinny cooking methods that add a surprising amount of flavor:

COOK ON A CEDAR PLANK: This is one of my favorite Skinny cooking secrets. It is a perfect way to roast vegetables, cook fish and prepare many other foods. The cedar adds a delicious taste and flavor to the meal, without adding a single calorie.

SAUTÉ: Sautéing with the smallest amount of extra virgin olive oil adds great flavor to your meat, fish or vegetables, including red peppers, snow peas, chicken, steak and salmon. Sautéing is a Skinny solution for making foods taste great with just a little added fat.

GRILLING: Grilling is another ideal Skinny cooking method and a great way to make over a meal. You can grill pizza, fish, beef, chicken, pork, veggies, fruit and potatoes. You can actually create an entire Skinny meal right on the grill! Grilling vegetables and fruit gives them a little face-lift and adds an excellent flavor, but no fat.

STOVETOP GRILL: If you don't have the space for a grill or don't like to grill in winter weather, consider using a grill pan to get similar results indoors. Paulette Mitchell, the author of

14 cookbooks, including *The Complete 15-Minute Gourmet: Creative Cuisine Fast and Fresh,* explains that cooking on a stovetop grill pan requires less oil than a skillet. Rather than pouring cooking oil into the grill pan, just lightly brush one side of the food to be cooked, such as chicken breasts, fish fillets or vegetables. Cook, oiled-side down. Brush the tops lightly with oil, turn and cook until done. Mitchell also recommends selecting a nonstick grill pan, which further reduces the amount of oil needed.

Check out Part Four: Skinny Cooking for additional Skinny cooking tips and techniques to try.

Try New Foods and Recipes

Trying a new food or recipe is a great way to make over your traditional meals. It's also a great way to discover different foods or recipes that you really like! In the summer, boost your intake of antioxidant-rich fruits and veggies and try new varieties of fresh local produce. In the winter—what I like to call cooking season—experiment in the kitchen with new recipes!

Slow Down and Enjoy

While you are trying new ways to make over your meal, make over your eating etiquette by slowing the speed at which you eat. It takes about 20 minutes for the brain to tell your body, *Hey there, I'm full—you can stop eating now.* So if you inhale dinner in five minutes and are grabbing seconds just a few minutes later because you think you are still hungry, the reality is that you don't even really know if you are still hungry because your body hasn't had time to tell you yet! Slow down, and truly enjoy the taste of what you are eating and the company you are eating with. Even try setting the utensils down between bites to help slow you down. 🆂🆁

<table>
<tr><td>SKINNY
RULE
14</td><td># Curb Your Cravings</td></tr>
</table>

Everyone gets cravings—most likely your cravings are driven by the taste of either salt or sugar. Right? But Skinny girls have a handful of tricks to satisfy their cravings without sacrificing their Skinny lifestyle. This is so important because salt is becoming known as a diet saboteur, a huge factor in your scale refusing to budge, and the majority of sugary foods are simply providing empty calories—minimal nutrition value.

The Nutrition Twins®, Tammy Lakatos Shames, RD, LD, CDN, CPT, and Lyssie Lakatos, RD, CDN, CPT, co-authors of *The Secret to Skinny,* offer surefire substitutes to quiet your next salt and/or sugar cravings. Instead of reaching for potato chips, pretzels or other salty snacks try:

- A celery stalk with 1 teaspoon of all-natural, unsalted peanut butter
- 3 cups unsalted, air-popped popcorn, seasoned with cayenne powder, onion powder, garlic powder, chili powder, coriander and cumin, or sprinkled with chili powder and paprika

And if it is candy that you crave, check out the Nutrition Twins® fruit substitutes below for any kind of candy that you love; they can give you nearly the same taste sensation and mouth feel, which will totally satisfy you. Best of all, fruit contains far less insulin-spiking sugar and is packed with fiber, so you'll feel fuller longer!

If you crave	Then you should eat
Chocolate	Fresh dates or figs rolled in cocoa powder (Portion guide: 4 dates, 2 large figs or 3 small figs)
Tangy sweets, such as Starburst, Skittles or Mike and Ike	Kiwi, pineapple or mango (Portion guide: 2 kiwi, ¾ cup chopped pineapple or ½ mango)
Tart candy, such as Smarties	Grapefruit, tart dried cherries or pomegranate (Portion guide: 1 small grapefruit, ¼ cup unsweetened tart dried cherries or ½ pomegranate)
Soft and gooey sweets, such as marshmallows, jelly beans or caramel	Fresh dates, dried apricots or dried plums (Portion guide: 4 dates, 4 dried apricots or 4 dried plums)
Pure sugar, such as cotton candy	Sugar-packed fruits, such as an overripe frozen banana or raisins (Portion guide: 1 small banana or ¼ cup raisins)

Here are a few of my personal favorite stand-ins to quiet a sweet tooth or assuage the craving for salt:

- Low-fat chocolate milk to kick a chocolate craving (Portion guide: 1 cup)
- Plain, low-fat Greek yogurt topped or drizzled with chocolate sauce and fruit to get rid of an ice cream craving (Portion guide: 1 cup yogurt and ½ cup chopped fruit)
- Walnuts or almonds toasted with garlic powder (Portion guide: 1 ounce [about 20–22 nuts])
- Hummus with sliced red peppers or cucumbers (Portion guide: 2 tablespoons of hummus and ½ cup sliced veggies)

Challenge yourself to use some of these tips and tricks to curb your next craving! And check out Skinny Rule #16 for tips on splurging every day! ⓢⓡ

SKINNY
RULE
15

Watch Your BLTs

No, not bacon, lettuce and tomato sandwiches... bites, licks and tastes! This helpful tip comes from a Skinny cousin of mine, Kristie Kinderman: Every bite, lick and taste adds up quickly when you're watching your calories. So think twice (and even three times) before you have that extra bite, lick or taste!

If you want to challenge yourself, try this fun little exercise. Keep a scrap of paper in your pocket for an entire day and every time you take an extra bite, lick or taste of something, jot it down. At the end of the day try to estimate how many extra calories piled up thanks to those little BLTs. To estimate how many calories are in a small amount of food, go to www.nutritiondata.com. It is an amazing online database of nutrition facts that lets you see how many calories are in different serving sizes of various foods. To start, go to the website and in the upper right-hand corner of the home page type in a food name and then click Search. You will quickly be able to see how many calories are approximately in a bite, lick or taste. Choose the one-ounce serving size from the drop-down menu for the food you've selected and it will give you a rough idea of how many calories were in that taste. Of course, depending on how many bites, licks and tastes of the food you had, the amount of calories will differ. And while I'm not calling you a big mouth, the calories may also vary depending on the size of your mouth!

This Skinny rule is especially important because people don't take the calories from those BLTs into account, but they do add up! Maybe it's a few extra bites while you're preparing dinner, followed by the lick of a spoon when you're cleaning up or a small taste off your friend's plate at a restaurant. Each of these seemingly innocent and perhaps even mindless acts adds calories. Controlling calorie intake is a delicate balance and nixing the extra bites, licks and tastes can and will make a difference in your weight.

Check out some approximate calories that come from just a small bite, lick or taste: 🅢🅡

Food	Approximate Calories from a Bite, Lick or Taste (based on a 1-ounce serving)
Lick of Peanut Butter	165
Lick of Frosting	116
Bite of Cake with Frosting	103
Few Bites of French Fries	93
Taste of Chicken Wing	60

SKINNY RULE 16 — Splurge Every Day

Could it really be true? A registered dietitian giving you permission—even encouraging you—to splurge every day? Believe it!

This Skinny rule is inspired by leading nutrition expert Elisa Zied, MS, RD, CDN, spokesperson for the American Dietetic Association and author of *Nutrition at Your Fingertips* and *Feed Your Family Right!* As she states, "I treat myself every day with a little bit of chocolate. I have it every day late in the morning, after I exercise."

This Skinny rule has helped Zied to lose weight and keep it off for more than a decade. Zied notes that chocolate helps her feel satisfied and she keeps the portion small. So what is considered a small portion of chocolate? Zied suggests aiming for a chocolate bar with 200 calories or less, and account for those calories as part of your daily eating routine.

> **Skinny Tip**
>
> As Brooke Shields told people.com, when she craves a chocolate fix she opts for the dark, nutrient-packed kind. Smart tip to try!

Here are some other decadent 200-calorie or less treats to splurge on:

- 1 cup of light vanilla ice cream
- 1 cup of chocolate pudding (made with fat-free milk)
- 1 ounce of cheddar cheese and a few pretzels
- 2 small handfuls of potato chips
- 1 chocolate chip cookie

This works for a couple of reasons. Number one: You are accounting for and factoring in the calories from your favorite treat. Number two: It helps to control your cravings, making you less likely to let your craving build up to an uncontrollable binge. This is where a lot of people go wrong. They think that because they're trying to eat healthy, they can't eat certain foods at all, and so deprive themselves. Yet think about it this way: If someone tells you that you can't have something, even if you didn't really want it in the first place, it suddenly becomes *so* desirable. It is this pattern that can set us up for trouble.

That is why it is your best Skinny bet to know what foods you crave—salty? sweet? sweet and salty?—and factor those foods into your eating routine. **SR**

<table>
<tr><td>

SKINNY
RULE
17

</td><td>

Enjoy Belly Laughs

</td></tr>
</table>

Could it be that Skinny people laugh more?

A 2005 study at Vanderbilt University Medical Center showed that laughing raised energy expenditure and increased heart rate by 10 to 20 percent. Better yet, laughing for 10 to 15 minutes a day could burn 10 to 40 calories a day. If you were to burn 40 calories every day by laughing, you'd burn 14,600 calories or about four pounds' worth over the course of a year! As the study's lead researcher, Maciej Buckowski, PhD, was quoted as saying, "People can't eat at McDonald's and then expect to laugh away their lunch." Although a good 15-minute laugh would burn up the calories in two Hershey's Kisses chocolate candies.

If you are reading this thinking that you don't even laugh for five minutes a day, challenge yourself to sneak in 15 minutes of laughter a day. One fun place to start is www.joke-of-the-day.com, which provides you with a free joke every day to get you laughing. Here is one from the site to start you off.

Angel's Food versus Devil's Food

In the beginning, God created the Heavens and the Earth and populated the Earth with broccoli, cauliflower and spinach, green and yellow and red vegetables of all kinds, so Man and Woman would live long and healthy lives.

Then using God's great gifts, Satan created Ben and Jerry's Ice Cream and Krispy Creme Donuts. And Satan said, "You want chocolate with that?"

And Man said, "Yes!" And Woman said, "And as long as you're at it, add some sprinkles." And they gained 10 pounds. And Satan smiled.

And God created healthful yogurt so that Woman might keep the figure that Man found so fair. And Satan brought forth white flour from the wheat, and sugar from the cane and combined them. And Woman went from size 6 to size 14.

So God said, "Try my fresh green salad." And Satan presented ranch dressing, buttery croutons and garlic toast on the side. And Man and Woman unfastened their belts following the repast.

God then said, "I have sent you heart-healthy vegetables and olive oil in which to cook them." And Satan brought forth deep-fried fish and chicken-fried steak so big it needed its own platter. And Man gained more weight and his cholesterol went through the roof.

God then created a light, fluffy white cake, named it "Angel Food Cake," and said, "It is good." Satan then created chocolate cake and named it "Devil's Food."

God then brought forth running shoes so that His children might lose those extra pounds. And Satan gave them cable TV with a remote control so Man would not have to toil changing the channels. And Man and Woman laughed and cried before the flickering blue light and gained even more pounds.

Then God brought forth the potato, naturally low in fat and brimming with nutrition. And Satan peeled off the healthful skin and sliced the starchy center into chips and deep-fried them. And Man gained still more pounds.

God then gave lean beef so that Man might consume fewer calories and still satisfy his appetite. And Satan created McDonald's and its 99-cent double cheeseburger. Then Satan said, "You want fries with that?" And Man replied, "Yes! And supersize them!" And Satan said, "It is good." And Man went into cardiac arrest.

God sighed and created quadruple-bypass surgery.

Then Satan created HMOs.

Make it one of your goals to laugh every day! **SR**

SKINNY RULE 18

Eat Like a Kid

W hen is the last time you had raisins for a snack? Had a peanut butter and jelly sandwich? Took a half hour to eat a meal? Or had someone saying to you: "You've already had enough juice today. Instead, you have to have milk" or "You have to drink milk with your dinner. Soda is just a treat." Most likely you enjoyed these kinds of foods or heard these lines or something similar as a kid, right? And if you have children, you've probably said some of these lines yourself!

Turns out, these are all good Skinny rules and eating more like a kid may be just the thing you need to live a Skinnier life.

Most kids follow a routine eating plan, with a sensible breakfast, lunch, dinner and snacks—just as Skinny people do! For the most part, children drink water, milk and only small amounts of juice. When it comes to sweets, kids enjoy them, but in small or moderate portion sizes and (as their parents and teachers are quick to remind them) sweets are just occasional treats. Kids tend to get pretty excited too, right? When is the last time you jumped for joy over a small taste of your favorite dessert?

Somewhere between grade school and the mortgage, all the Skinny habits you used to follow as a child shifted, transformed and flew out the window. Remember when your day started with a delicious and nutritious breakfast of cereal with milk and a small glass of watered-down orange juice? That wholesome breakfast got replaced with a jumbo mug of coffee filled with cream and sugar to fuel you through lunch. You grab lunch from the most convenient location, not necessarily a healthy lunch, accompanied by a 20-ounce (or bigger) cup of some sugar-laden or fizzy diet drink, stop by a vending machine for a snack full of empty calories and then end the day with dinner at a time when you would have likely already been asleep as a child.

It's clear that acting more like a kid will help keep your weight down and ultimately help you lead a healthier life.

Here are some fun ways to start:

START EACH DAY with a nutritious, balanced breakfast—not from a drive-thru and not just a cup of coffee.

PACK A LUNCH with a balanced formula, like a peanut butter and jelly sandwich, a piece of fruit, a bag of carrot sticks, a small treat and a cup of low-fat or nonfat milk.

DRINK MOSTLY WATER and low-fat or nonfat milk and have 100 percent fruit juice occasionally. Of course, water the juice down to dilute it. (For more adult tastes, try a refreshing juice spritzer with half club soda and half juice.)

SNACK ON HEALTHY FOODS you would have had as a kid, like fruits, dried fruits, vegetables, whole-grain crackers and cheese sticks.

GET TOGETHER A GAME of pickup basketball, soccer, tag or some other fun outdoor activity with friends or a group of kids and adults. **SR**

SKINNY RULE 19	Downsize Your Bowl

Registered dietitian and nutrition expert Lisa Young, author of *The Portion Teller,* says it best: "People need to be less concerned about what they're eating and more concerned about how much they are eating." This is absolutely true. Although it may seem surprising, overeating is simply overeating, whether you're eating salad or a dozen cookies.

One easy Skinny trick to follow is to downsize your bowl. Seems too simple to work? Research has proven that bowl size actually makes a big impact on portion size! Brian Wansink, director of the Cornell food and brand lab, conducted a study to determine how bowl size impacted portion size, and published the results in the *American Journal of Preventive Medicine.* He had 85 graduate students and nutrition science professors (people who definitely know the importance of portion control!) attend an ice cream social and the attendees were given either a medium (17 ounces) or large (34 ounces) ice cream bowl and a medium (2 ounces) or large (3 ounces) ice cream scoop. The experts who had the large ice cream dishes served themselves 31 percent more ice cream! The combination of the large dish plus the large scoop resulted in an even more dramatic result—a 53 percent larger serving than the group given the medium bowls and medium scoops.

The lesson here is clear: Downsize your bowl. Not only for ice cream but for other foods, too, like cereal, pasta, potatoes…you get the idea. If you swap the large bowl for a smaller-sized bowl, the portion will *look* more filling, as Wansink determined, and will also help you to serve yourself less.

Attached to your big bowl? Another way to downsize your portion size is to fill up the bowl with lower-calorie foods so that you eat less of the high-calorie stuff. The next time you want ice cream, fill a bowl with fresh fruit, like strawberries and blueberries, and then top the fruit with a small amount of ice cream. Instead of a bowl of tortilla chips, fill a bowl with crunchy celery slices and black bean chips (a smarter choice because they have belly-filling fiber), then dip the chips and celery into a bowl of chunky salsa, which is filling and low in calories. (There are only 8 calories in 2 tablespoons of salsa—you can have a whole cup for under 70 calories.)

Every little way you shave calories takes you a step closer to living a Skinnier life! 🆂🆁

Two

Skinny Fitness

| SKINNY RULE 20 | Be Selfish |

Have you ever woken up and thought, How in the world did it get to be Friday already? Let's face it: Life moves forward at a dizzying pace and if you don't get selfish with your time, week after week can speed by and exercise is one of the things that gets lost in the shuffle.

Many Skinny people don't even realize it, but they are selfish when it comes to their exercise. After all, Skinny people are just as bogged down with busy schedules as the rest of us, but they make exercise a priority in their lives. In fact, the National Weight Control Registry, which tracks a group of people who have lost 30 pounds or more and kept it off for at least one year, shows that 90 percent of successful dieters exercise for an average of one hour a day.

What does this being selfish tip really mean? It means making time in your busy life for exercise. Keep in mind that what exercise is right for you will vary from person to person. For some it may be running every day; for others it may be running around with their kids on the playground; and for still others it may be playing their favorite sport. At the end of the day, the key to Skinny success is taking the time to do it!

So if you're looking at your schedule and can't figure out where to squeeze in exercise, be selfish and schedule in time to work out. Think of it as setting a daily appointment for yourself! **SR**

SKINNY
RULE
21

Try Yoga—A Skinny Secret of Celebs

How do Skinny celebs and pro athletes stay in top shape? Their Skinny secret is yoga, an exercise that is known for sculpting lean, sexy muscle. To practice the balance of body, mind and spirit, many celebrities and professional athletes turn to yoga instructor Mark Blanchard. Actor Andy Garcia notes that Mark's workouts are "the most intense workout I've ever done. It improved my strength, flexibility and my golf game."

YOGA literally means, "to join or yoke together," which brings the body, mind and spirit together into one harmonious experience. There are hundreds of types of yoga. Here is a breakdown of a few of the different types of yoga, as defined by the American Yoga Association:

HATHA YOGA: This combination of physical movements and postures, with breathing techniques, is what most people associate with yoga practice.

RAJA YOGA: Incorporates exercise and breathing practice with meditation and study; called the "royal road."

KARMA YOGA: This type of yoga is based on the philosophy that all movement and work of any kind is done with the mind centered on a personal concept of God.

While there are eight steps of classical yoga, as noted by the American Yoga Association, most modern Western yoga classes focus on asana, physical exercises; pranayama, breathing techniques; and pratyahara, preparation for meditation. Research on the health benefits of yoga has brought it to the forefront of preventive health practices, so much so that even physicians recommend yoga practice to patients at risk of heart disease, as well as those with back pain, arthritis, depression and other chronic conditions.

Blanchard explains that it can be confusing and daunting to figure out if yoga is right for you and which form of yoga is right for you. He suggests that if you have tried one yoga class and didn't like it, don't give up! Yoga is like any other workout: It really depends on the class and the type of workout. "Many people don't realize that you don't have to be flexible to do yoga. You don't have to have a quiet mind and chant to do yoga. Yoga is not a religion and yoga can be cardiovascular and can be an intense workout," states Blanchard.

One woman explains that she was able to slim down in just four weeks by doing Mark's True Power Yoga DVD or class five times a week. In that time she lost 15 pounds and 12 percent of her body fat. As she said, "I feel stronger. My stomach is flatter and my arms and butt are toned. My back pain is gone, my mood is improved, and I have a sense of calm." 🆂🆁

SKINNY RULE 22 · Try These Top Celebrity Workouts

Meg Ryan, Reese Witherspoon, Christian Slater and Dennis Quaid are just a few of the celebrities who work out with personal trainer Michael George. To find out how they maintain their Skinny figures, I asked Michael for the exercises that keep these celebs in top shape. Check out these moves and try to incorporate them into your workout routine.

Meg Ryan routinely does walking lunges with bicep curls. Michael George advises doing two sets of 15 to 25 repetitions, three times a week.

Reese Witherspoon does a traditional yoga move called sun salutations. This is a series of yoga poses moving from downward dog into plank, then back into downward dog and ending in standing pose. Michael George recommends adding one set of three sun salutations, three times a week, to your workout routine.

Or you could get in a little boxing or kicking with a heavy punching bag or boxing mitts, as Christian Slater does. Try this for 10 to 20 minutes, three times a week, per Michael George.

Do you remember doing squat thrusts—the exercise where you squat, kick your legs out behind you to get into a push-up position and then jump back up? You likely did them in gym class when you were younger. Michael George works this traditional move into Dennis Quaid's workout routine. Try one set of 5 to 10 repetitions, three times a week, according to Michael George.

Last but not least, Michael George gets all his clients doing light jogging to brisk walking for 20 to 40 minutes, three to four times a week. 🅢🅡

| SKINNY
RULE
23 | **Make Exercise a Habit** |

Think about everything you do on a daily basis as part of your routine—brushing your teeth, showering, putting on clothes, eating meals. Now imagine if you cut out one of those daily acts to save time. What if you showed up to work and everyone you spoke to had awful morning breath? Start thinking of exercise as just as important to starting your day as brushing your teeth. As celebrity trainer Gunnar Peterson told CNN, "Get on a regular routine. Exercise should be a cornerstone of your life, like brushing your teeth. It's not even an option to blow it off."

To stick with a workout routine that works, think of making exercise an essential part of your routine. A recent study in the *European Journal of Social Psychology* of 96 people who were interested in forming a new habit, such as eating a piece of fruit with lunch or doing a 15-minute run each day, found that it takes anywhere from 18 to 254 days to form a new habit. The age-old advice of 21 days to form a habit was blown out of the water with this study. What the study markedly found is that some habits take much longer than others to form. For example, a habit of adding 15 minutes of exercise before breakfast each morning took much longer to form than a habit of increasing water consumption or adding a piece of fruit to the diet.

Skinny people make exercise part of their routine and life—a habit. Instead of going out to eat with friends or to a movie every week, they join an exercise class, a hiking club or a soccer team. In a one-hour exercise class you will burn about 350 calories.[†] Instead of going out for heavy meals or beers, Skinny girls go dancing on a night on the town. Going out dancing for just one hour will burn about 300 calories,[†] as opposed to sitting on a barstool, which will burn few, if any, calories. Not to mention all the calories you'll be drinking if you are plunked down on a barstool.

Skinny people also stay on the move. A study by the Endocrine Research Unit of the Mayo Clinic found that Skinny people tend to move around more. Next time you're calling a friend, walk around while you're talking, or instead of sitting and watching your favorite television program, use it as an opportunity to exercise. Try keeping free weights or a balance ball in your television room as an easy-to-grab option for exercise. Lifting weights during a 30-minute television program will burn about 204 calories.[†]

[†]   Based on a 150-pound person.

Other simple ways to stay Skinny by moving and making exercise part of your life: Make an exercise appointment with yourself, dust off your bike and try using it as a mode of transportation to run an errand or even just to go for a ride. 🅢🅡

SKINNY
RULE
24

Sneak It In

Sneaking exercise into your regular routine is a powerful Skinny secret. Even 10-minute bouts of exercise seem to be effective in reducing waist size and body mass index (BMI). And, as all Skinny girls know, it's much easier to find an extra 10 minutes in a schedule than figuring out how to squeeze in 30 minutes or more of exercise.

Why does this Skinny rule work? It creates consistency with exercise because 10 minutes is an easy-to-digest time to get moving and keep moving. Another powerful component to the 10-minute bursts of exercise is that once you get moving for just 10 minutes, it becomes motivation to keep moving longer. And, of course, the more you move the more calories you burn, and the more calories you burn the Skinnier you'll be!

Think about your schedule for a few minutes and see if you can find ways to sneak in just 10-minute bursts of exercise. Here are some quick ways to get moving:

- Go for a brisk walk.
- Grab a set of hand weights (go easy if you haven't lifted weights before or if you're just getting started).
- Try a few yoga poses.
- Park your car a 10-minute walk away from work or from the mall.
- Bike instead of driving.

When can you sneak in 10 minutes? Instead of hitting the snooze button, exercise before you shower in the morning. Take part of your lunch break to exercise. Add a walk to your commute home from work. Exercise during commercials while you are watching television, or even at night before bed.

What can you sneak in? Raking the lawn (49 calories per 10 minutes), sit-ups (91 calories per 10 minutes), jogging in place (90 calories per 10 minutes), jumping rope (113 calories per 10 minutes), brisk walk (43 calories per 10 minutes), lifting weights (34 calories per 10 minutes).[†]

Even if that doesn't sound like a lot of calories to burn, jogging in place burns 90 calories more than you would have just sitting on your tush! And burning those extra 90 calories even just one time a day is equal to a grand total of 32,850 calories a year, which is equal to burning up about nine pounds! 🆂🆁

| SKINNY RULE **25** | Do It at Home |

D o you know someone who signed up for a pricey gym membership, went for a while and then wound up paying the monthly fee but didn't go to the gym at all? Statistics show that about 90 percent of people who join health and fitness clubs stop going within the first 90 days. This can end up being a huge waste of money—and it doesn't help you reach your Skinny goals at all!

While working out at home comes with its own price tag, it can definitely have its advantages. The best part about

---

[†]   Based on a 150-pound person.

working out at home is that your workout space can't get any more convenient. After a long day at work, school or home with the kids, you can quickly slip on your gym shoes, roll out your yoga mat or pull out your weights and start sweating in no time at all.

Supplying your workout space can range from simple to elaborate. To start, equip your space with hand weights. Opt for a set of hand weights with a range of weights—for example, 5, 7½ and 10 pounds. Or, if you need to start even lighter, buy one set of light hand weights (1 or 2 pounds) and add to your set as your strength increases. How do you know what weight to start with? You should be able to do at least three sets of 12 repetitions of an exercise without feeling strained. When you are done with the three sets, your muscles will feel tired, but you should not feel as though you are overstressing your body. Every workout space needs a comfortable yoga-style mat, too, which is perfect for doing push-ups, crunches, yoga, stretching and other core-building moves.

Working out with fitness DVDs is another great way to switch around your workouts while still in the comfort of your home. Check out some of my favorite DVDs in Appendix B: Skinny Tools. ⑤

| SKINNY RULE 26 | Find Your Skinny Exercise Solution |

Exercise can take many different shapes and forms—it's definitely not one size fits all. When *People* asked superfit Brooke Shields what she does to stay in such great shape, she laughed and said, "I'm a closet superhero!" Her real Skinny secret is a combination of yoga and spinning and staying away from weights. Whether you need to channel your inner superhero, start doing yoga or get on a bike, finding the winning formula that is unique to you is key. And what works for you may be different than what works for the next person. Here is the inside scoop on what celebrities shared with www.fitnessmagazine.com about exercise routines.

Britney Spears whipped herself back into shape for her Circus tour by dancing to her choreographed hip-hop moves. As Dave Van Daff, senior director of education and development for Bally Total Fitness, explained to www.fitnessmagazine.com, dancing is considered to be a high-intensity cardio workout and "burns high amounts of calories and body fat." Kristi Yamaguchi left the pro tour in 2002 to start a family. When the world champ and Olympic gold medalist in figure skating needed to tone up to slip into the slinky outfits on *Dancing with the Stars,* Pilates worked for her. She explains, "It's about building your core, getting it strong, because everything radiates from there. But I've found that you can use it to work all the muscles in your body. And since you're not doing a lot of reps, you're maintaining a lean look." The key is that each celebrity mentioned above has her own formula, which works for her. If you are trying to figure out what is the best formula for you and have no idea where to start, try one of the exercises mentioned above—yoga, spinning, Pilates or dancing. If you belong to a gym or fitness center, explore the different classes they offer. Who knows? You might just find *your* Skinny exercise solution. 🆂🆁

SKINNY RULE 27

Pump It Up

When you think about pumping it up, you likely think of bulging muscles and outrageously heavy weights. While that may be good if you're looking to bulk up, to sculpt lean, Skinny muscle, choose light weights or resistance bands and do more repetitions.

Why is pumping it up such an important part of a Skinny exercise routine? Lifting weights helps to build muscle. Although muscle weighs more than body fat, it takes up less space than fat (you can weigh more but wear a smaller size) and is metabolically active, meaning it *burns* calories while you are sitting still. This helps big time: The more calories your body burns the better and, some may argue, the easier it is to maintain a healthy weight. There are other health perks that come with lifting weights, too. Perhaps the most notable is that weight-bearing exercise helps you build strong bones, an important factor in preventing osteoporosis.

Rich and Helene Guzman, the co-owners of L.A. R.O.X and trainers to Hilary Swank, told www.fitnessmagazine.com that Swank gained 19 pounds of muscle for her role in *Million Dollar Baby.* The routine included doing a muscle-building strength routine two to three times a week. The exercises all use resistance bands or tubing. In addition, you'll need a step bench or stairs and a chair or stability ball. Try these exercises to get buff arms like Hilary Swank, courtesy of www.fitnessmagazine.com:

CHEST FLYE: Tie a resistance band or tubing around a sturdy object at about chest height. Stand facing away from the anchor point, holding one end of the band in each hand with your feet apart and arms out to the sides, palms facing forward. Slowly bring the ends of the band together in front of your chest, rotating your palms down. Slowly return to start, keeping your elbows slightly bent; repeat. Do as many reps as you can without sacrificing form.

TRICEPS EXTENSION: Untie the band and place one end under your right foot, holding the other end in your right hand. Raise your right arm next to your head, keeping elbow bent and close to your ear. Slowly extend your arm, then lower to start and repeat. Do as many reps as you can. Switch sides.

BICEPS CURL: Stand on the center of the band, feet shoulder-width apart. Hold one end of the band in each hand, palms facing up and elbows close to your sides. Keeping your elbows pressed into your rib cage, slowly curl your hands toward your shoulders, keeping your wrists straight. Lower and repeat. Do as many reps as you can.

Trainers recommend doing strength training two to three times a week with cardio on the same or alternate days. For the cardio component, aim for at least 30 minutes of jogging, elliptical training, walking, cycling or swimming. **SR**

SKINNY
RULE
28

Play the Pounds Away

Okay, I've managed to get through quite a few tips on exercise without bringing up the fact that most people just flat out hate to exercise. It's time to address this and provide Skinny solutions for those who truly despise exercise.

Try shifting your thought process about exercise and think more like a kid, because instead of thinking about exercise as something they have to do, kids enjoy doing it! Kids tend to be really active, too. Playing on sports teams, playing with friends, going outside on the playground at school—kids are always looking for ways to burn their energy. And even though few offices designate recess during the lunch hour, it's just as important for adults. Dr. Jamie Laubisch of Johns Hopkins Medical Center suggests that this kind of break is especially important when you are busy, and explains that playing with your kids definitely counts as exercise.

Linda Quinn, registered dietitian, explains that part of the solution is changing the way you think about exercise. "Think about the terminology. I have to go 'work out.' Instead, think: I am going out to play. I like to feel young every day by acting young. Play is one activity that separates children from adults. Be more childlike, and you will feel and look years younger."

Quinn adds, "I play almost every day after work and double on the weekend" and credits playing for her Skinny physique. If she's not at a park Rollerblading, then she's riding her bike along the Erie Canal in upstate New York. Rather than thinking about how many calories she's burned or how long she's been exercising, she just enjoys herself: "I revel at all the different birds, fish, turtles, snakes, muskrats, raccoons, beavers and deer that I see along the way. Sometimes I get so wrapped up in the osprey that I see along the trail I forget I just rode 20 miles."

Playing is a perfect way to connect with your body and nature—and get healthy in the process. Instead of scheduling time for a workout, work in playtime for yourself. When you say you're going to "play," it quickly becomes something you want to do, rather than a chore that you have to do each day. What counts as play? Anything that gets you up and moving! Biking, swimming, kayaking, surfing, hiking, Rollerblading, skateboarding, exploring nature trails—any activity you enjoy. During the week, playtime will be more limited, but you can enjoy bigger adventures on the weekends when you have more time.

The other great thing about playing is that you design the route and set the goals—no one else. This is perfect for someone who isn't in a routine of exercising and needs to be "playing" more often. You can start with a short play session, like trying a 10-minute bike ride or a 10-minute nature walk. Then the next time you "play," the length can increase and before you know it you will be finding ways to extend your "playtime" rather than figuring out how you can get out of doing it. Another fun option is to join an adult league or a team of your favorite sport. You can easily find an adult swim team, soccer team, running club or ice hockey team in your city.

How are you going to play today? 🆂🆁

SKINNY RULE 29

Invest in Yourself

Regardless of how you are investing your money in stocks, bonds or your 401(k) plan, there is one place that you must invest in on a routine basis— yourself! You are given one and only one body to last you for the rest of your life and that makes investing in yourself one of the most important investments you will ever make. And exercise is one of the best ways to invest in your body.

How do you go about it? More important than spending money on equipment that may just end up collecting dust is investing in the time out of your busy life to exercise. Without investing in the time to exercise, the gym membership, new bikes, treadmills, weights, yoga mats and the like will all wind up being a poor investment. It is an absolute *must* to carve out the time to exercise.

I am the mom of two boys, ages three and one. I run my own consulting business, and I am writing this book. I definitely know what it feels like to be pressed for time (or extra energy) for exercise. But I have to do it, so it is an investment that I make almost every day. So no excuses! Take a good, hard look at your schedule and figure out how you can start investing in yourself by making the time to exercise.

There are several pieces of equipment that can make exercise more enjoyable, comfortable and convenient. Here are some that may be worth investing in to make your exercise experience better:

SNEAKERS: The most important piece of "equipment" is a good pair of sneakers. Almost all types of exercise that you do will require a comfortable, well-fitting pair of sneakers. Believe it or not, sneakers get worn out and need replacing before they look like they do; at a minimum, replace your sneakers every six months. The insides of your sneakers get a tremendous workout, so replacing your sneakers is key to staying comfortable while you're exercising. If you would like to learn more about sneakers, check out www.runnersworld.com for everything from a guide to knowing what type of arch you have to seeing comparisons of the latest sneaker types and finding out from the experts which sneakers are really worth paying for.

BICYCLE: Another piece of exercise gear that I personally think everyone should own is a bicycle. Biking is a great form of exercise—plus, it's a family-friendly activity. In addition, biking feels more like playing than exercising. If you live in a bike-friendly community, you can use your new wheels to get from here to there; you will save on gas, burn calories and help the environment all at the same time! Bikes can cost anywhere from a few hundred bucks to thousands. Consult your local bike shop about what type of bike is right for you. Don't forget to bike safely and invest in a good helmet, too.

GADGETS: There are many exercise gadgets that are relatively inexpensive and do not take up too much room. Among those to invest in are an exercise band, a medicine ball, a stability ball and a yoga mat. These are gadgets you can rely on to bring your workout routine to a higher level.

GLIDE AWAY: Pick up a pair of Rollerblades, ice skates or roller skates. All three types of exercise will burn calories and firm up legs and butt muscles.

PERSONAL TRAINER: Working out with a personal trainer is an important option to consider when creating your investment strategy for exercise. A personal trainer can help to design a workout plan that will yield the results you are looking for and is worth every penny!

As far as other ways to invest in your exercise routine, the options are almost endless. My biggest word of advice would be to carefully examine what you are buying and determine if you are really going to use it. Avoid buying the gadget on the 3:00 a.m. infomercial that sounds too good to be true, because it probably *is* too good to be true.

Like other investments, create a strategy. If you have nothing at home right now, that is okay. Examine how much space you have to dedicate to exercise equipment. If you're tight on space, stick to easy-to-store items like sneakers, hand weights, a yoga mat and a medicine ball. If you have a bit more space, save up for some bigger pieces of equipment, like your very own bike. Have fun creating your exercise equipment plan and investing in your health! ⑤®

| SKINNY RULE 30 | Train Like a Pro Athlete |

I work with professional athletes, which is both a challenge and very rewarding. Specifically, I counsel the Ottawa and Binghamton Senators (NHL and AHL) hockey teams. What I have learned firsthand in working with pro athletes is that while they do have a distinct and inborn talent for their sport, they also possess an incredible work ethic. In the world of professional sports, although players are technically only "in season" for a portion of the year, the reality is that they are training non-stop, year-round.

How does this relate to you? You, too, can be a step closer to working out like professional athletes by adopting their work ethic when it comes to your own exercise routine. So no excuses: Think like a professional athlete and make getting a workout into your routine a priority and an essential part of your day. A Skinny lifestyle isn't a part-time, one-season sport: You need to commit to it every day, year-round, in order to see sustained results.

In addition to consistency, we can learn from the way pro athletes vary their training. I mostly consult with professional hockey players. While they spend a majority of their time on the ice, they spend considerable time off the ice doing cross training. You can use this philosophy to your advantage, too. Say tennis is your sport of choice. Rather than just playing tennis, you should alternate your workouts and add off-the-court workouts into your weekly routine. Cross training could include jogging, agility work-outs to improve your speed, shoulder exercises to improve your shoulder strength and so on. If you are not sure what specific types of cross-training exercises would best benefit your sport or exercise of choice, talk with a personal trainer who could set up a cross-training program for you. You will definitely see the benefits in your sports performance.

Last but not least, the players adopt the philosophy that nutrition makes a difference in performance. Players have specific pregame meals, postgame refueling strategies, daily eating plans and, perhaps most important, focus on staying adequately hydrated. Throughout this book, I have offered tips on getting enough fluids, but there are even more specific guidelines when it comes to staying hydrated for work-ing out. Hydration is key because by the time your brain signals thirst, you are already 1 percent underhydrated and by the time you are 2 percent underhydrated your perfor-mance will decrease by 7 to 10 percent or more!

Professional athletes start their workouts well hydrated. You need to go into your workout well hydrated and the best way to do that is to drink at least eight cups of water every day. Then, above and beyond that, you should be hav-ing about four to six ounces of water every 15 to 20 minutes during exercise. This is equal to about four to six big gulps of fluid.

Now a quick word on what to drink. Many pro ath-letes use specialized drinks during workouts, which their bodies need because of the length of time they are work-ing out. Yet, unless you are working out longer than an hour, remember that plain water will do the trick! If you are working out consistently for longer than an hour, then switch to a sports drink like Gatorade to fuel tired muscles. You may be thinking, Don't these drinks have a lot of sugar? The answer is yes, but it is for a purpose. Sports drinks are designed to deliver the body carbohydrates in a 6 percent carbohydrate blend, which is the scientifically determined amount of carbohydrates that the body needs to fuel exercise. As an added bonus, they include electrolytes that aid in maintaining fluid balance. Most important, remember that sports drinks are not needed for a casual walk around the block but would be a performance booster for a two-hour-long weekend bike ride.

These are just guidelines, as fluid needs actually vary greatly from person to person, depending on how much you sweat and workout conditions. If you're curious about how much is right for you, hop on the scale before your next workout. Then immediately after, check your weight again. If you are losing weight during exercise, you need to ramp up the amount of fluid that you are drinking and aim to keep weight loss during exercise to less than one pound. The rule of thumb is this: For every pound of weight you lose during exercise, you need to refuel with 16 to 24 ounces of water. Why? Because, I am sorry to say, the weight that you are losing is water weight and not true weight loss. It is crucial to replenish your system after exercise if you are losing weight during your workouts.

Follow these tips and you, too, can be a step closer to working out like a pro! ⑤ℛ

SKINNY
RULE
31

Keep It Interesting

Maybe you have worked out consistently in the past or perhaps you even are doing so now, but you feel as if you are in a rut or even just plain bored with exercise. Keeping interested in working out is a Skinny secret.

What you love to do may change over time and with the seasons. That's a good thing for your body. Over time your body becomes accustomed to doing a certain type and amount of exercise, making variety a key ingredient to living a Skinny life. Let's say you walk four miles a few times a week. A great achievement. But over time, your body will become accustomed to this and in order to keep losing weight or maintaining your weight, you will have to ramp it up.

One of the best ways to keep up your interest level is to consult with a personal trainer. A trainer can help you figure out a workout or "play" routine that is right for you, and that is key when starting or reworking an exercise regimen.

Lots of Skinny girls work out with personal trainers, whether for every workout or for an occasional training session. If it works with your budget and you can afford regular appointments with a personal trainer, go for it! But if you're like most of the world (myself included), that may break the bank. Instead, schedule a few appointments with a personal trainer who will show you exercises to do with the equipment you have at home or at the gym, like hand weights, a balance ball, a medicine ball and the like. Then you can apply the tips you've learned when you work out on your own. What is great about working out with a personal trainer is that he can teach you new exercises, instruct you on using the proper form (so you don't wind up injuring yourself) and even introduce you to new exercise equipment. When searching for a personal trainer, make sure he is certified by a reputable organization like the American College of Sports Medicine (ACSM) or the American Council on Exercise (ACE), and that he isn't just a fly-by-night or self-proclaimed personal trainer.

So consider a personal trainer when creating your investment strategy for exercise. It is an important option to weigh and in most cases is worth every penny!

If you don't have the extra cash to spare for a personal

trainer or just are not sure that's the right approach for you, hop on the Internet and search for inspiring training routines that you can pick up free of charge. One of my favorite Skinny websites is www.fitnessmagazine.com. Here is a No-Fail Cardio Plan designed by Jeanette Jenkins, founder of the Hollywood Trainer for her client, Queen Latifah. It is designed to blast away 350 calories in 35 minutes! The workout uses RPE, or Rate of Perceived Exertion from a scale of 1 to 10 to determine your speed. Check out more information below on RPE if you have never used it to gauge your workouts before. It's an awesome Skinny tool. Here is the workout from www.fitnessmagazine.com:

Minutes	Pace	RPE
0:00–5:00	Warm up	5
5:00–7:00	Begin to intensify	6–7
7:00–11:00	Maintain steady pace	7
11:00–12:00	Sprint, 1 minute	8–9
12:00–14:00	Recover, lower intensity	6–7
14:00–15:30	Sprint, 90 seconds	8–9
15:30–17:30	Recover, lower intensity	6–7
17:30–19:15	Sprint, 1 minute and 45 seconds	8–9
19:15–21:15	Recover, lower intensity	6–7
21:15–23:15	Sprint, 2 minutes	8–9
23:15–25:30	Recover, lower intensity	6–7
25:30–30:30	Gradual acceleration (increase speed by 10% each minute)	8–9
30:30–35:00	Cool down	5

What is the Rate of Perceived Exertion (RPE)? A scale based on the research of Gunnar Borg to help gauge how intensely you are working out. There are different versions of the scale but the 10-point version is what the above workout was based on; in my opinion, that is the easiest one to use. What is best about the RPE scale is that you can use it to tailor workouts to your own fitness level, since what constitutes a "5" for you may be different from what someone else considers to be a "5." Adapt this scale to other workouts that you do: 0 = nothing at all; 0.5 = very, very light; 1 = very light; 2 = fairly light; 3 = moderate; 4 = somewhat hard; 5 = hard; 7 = very hard; 10 = very, very hard (max). 🆂🆁

SKINNY
RULE
32

Be Consistent

Celebrity trainer Michael George says it best: "Consistency and moderation are the keys to weight management for life." There is more to come on moderation in Part Three: Skinny Foods, but in the meantime, let's talk about consistency with exercise. George shared a secret of his: When time is tight, he breaks his exercise time into 3-, 10- or 20-minute workouts, allowing him to be consistent with his exercise routine while adjusting his workouts for his busy days.

This is a great way to keep from allowing an overscheduled life to turn into an excuse not to exercise. So many times I hear people saying (and even catch myself saying sometimes), I just don't have the time to exercise. The reality is that everyone's life is busy—just in different ways. My life is busy with parenting two little guys and running a business. Others' lives may be hectic because of work schedules, their children's schedules, caring for an aging parent.... No matter how complicated your life is, take a look at your schedule and figure out a way to make exercise a consistent fixture in your lifestyle. Whether you get up an hour earlier to work out before the day starts; squeeze in a walk, bike ride, jog or exercise class during lunch; hit the gym while the kids are at soccer practice; or hit the treadmill after the kids have gone to sleep, figure out a time that works for you so you can keep to a consistent workout schedule. And on days when timing is especially tight, aim for a 10- or 15-minute workout instead of a longer one—staying consistent is key.

Keeping consistent also means constantly reevaluating your schedule. What works for you during the fall may be different than what works for you during the spring because schedules are always changing. **SR**

SKINNY RULE **33**	Record It and Track It

J ust as it's important to keep track of what you eat, it's important—and motivating—to keep track of your exercise routine.

My husband, Bill, tracks his workout mileage with an online tracking tool and credits it as a key motivator in keeping him exercising. He uses www.mapmyride.com to keep track of how many miles he logs on a daily, weekly and monthly basis and, perhaps even more important, how many calories he burns. Mapmyride.com focuses on cycling, yet it allows you to record other types of exercise, too, like running, hiking, a gym workout, basketball and so on. You can even save typical routes that you run or bike, and then just plug them into your training log. There is a similar site, geared more toward runners, called www.mapmyrun.com.

These types of tools are perfect additions to your arsenal of exercise tools. In addition to tracking your mileage, they offer ways to track your weight and body mass index. You can even add training goals and participate in challenges, like running 100 miles in 30 days.

If you become a paying member of the website, you can have access to training plans like First-time Marathoner Training Plan, an 18-week training regimen to get you in shape for a marathon. So the website can double as your very own virtual personal trainer as well! If you're not into technology, no worries! Start a separate exercise calendar to record your daily exercise. Look for a free one from your bank or another local organization. Then keep it in an easy-to-reach location, so you can quickly update it after your daily workouts.

The sites mentioned in this section are just two examples of online resources, although there are many other similar options out there. Seek out which one is right for you or use the good old pen and paper method! 🆂🆁

| SKINNY RULE **34** | Get to the Heart of the Matter |

Monitoring your heart rate is a Skinny secret to determining how intensely you are working out and getting the most out of your workout. This trick is especially helpful if you are new to exercising, so that you can better determine how hard you're making your heart work and how hard you should work it. Monitoring your heart rate helps you customize your workouts and can help you burn up stored fat more effectively.

One way to calculate your target heart rate(s) is to use the Karvonen Formula, which is the gold standard used by organizations like the American College of Sports Medicine, to calculate heart rate goals. Even though it looks tricky, don't shy away from it. It's actually pretty simple. Ready to get started? Read on!

FIRST, calculate your resting heart rate. Take a big, deep breath and if you're not relaxed, sit back, close your eyes and relax for a few minutes. Using your pointer and middle fingers, apply light pressure to the backside of your wrist or the pulse point under your chin by your neck to find your pulse. If you don't feel your pulse at first, lightly search around until you feel it. Now count how many beats you feel in 10 seconds. Multiply that number by six and that will give you your approximate pulse for a minute and your resting heart rate, which you'll need for the equation below.

SECOND, calculate your maximum heart rate:

$$220 - (age) = \text{Max Heart Rate}$$

THIRD, calculate your heart rate reserve (you will need this number for the next part of the formula):

$$\text{Max Heart Rate} - \text{Resting Heart Rate} = \text{Heart Rate Reserve (HRR)}$$

FOURTH, using your resting heart rate number and your HRR number, follow the equations below to determine your low- and high-intensity target heart rates:

$$\text{HRR} \times 50\% = \underline{\quad} + \text{Resting Heart Rate} = \text{Low-Intensity Target Heart Rate}$$

> HRR x 80% = ___ + Resting Heart Rate
> = High-Intensity Target Heart Rate

For example, a 40-year-old with a resting heart rate of 70:

> 220 – 40 = Max Heart Rate of 180

> Max Heart Rate of 180
> – Resting Heart Rate of 70 = HRR of 110

> (110 x 50%) + 70 = Low-Intensity
> Target Heart Rate of 125

> (110 x 80%) + 70 = High-Intensity
> Target Heart Rate of 158

Now you can use these numbers to your advantage. Moderate- to vigorous-intensity exercise is needed for weight loss, meaning that during your workouts you should be exerting yourself toward the upper end of your target heart rate.

Not into math? The Mayo Clinic has a great tool that does the calculation for you. Check it out at www.mayoclinic.com/health/target-heart-rate/SM00083. If all these numbers are too much for you, there is a simpler way to figure out how intensively you are working out. You know you are working out at a moderate to vigorous intensity when it becomes difficult to talk due to the exertion of exercise. If you can carry on a conversation easily, you need to step it up to get closer to your high-intensity target heart rate. 🆂🆁

SKINNY RULE 35

Learn to Love Exercise!

Take a cue from Skinny girl Ashley Tisdale, star of *High School Musical,* who shared her Skinny secrets with *People* magazine. She explained that making time for the gym once "felt like torture." Her Skinny tip to get motivated? "Now before I work out," she says, "I think, 'I love exercise'—and it works." Finding your own workout mantra can get you in the right frame of mind for sticking to an exercise plan. Try these Skinny mantras and choose one that is right for you:

- Exercise will give me more energy.
- No excuses…I can do it.
- Exercise will help my clothes fit better.
- Exercise will make me strong and lean.
- I will enjoy this workout and feel great afterwards.

Take a few moments and think about what types of exercise you love. Running? Skiing? Playing soccer? Hiking? Riding a bike? Doing yoga? Swimming? Walking? Dancing? Lifting weights? Now when is the last time you did that?

Learning to love exercise or choosing an exercise you already enjoy is one of the most powerful Skinny rules there is. Consistent exercisers will tell you that they love the exercise they choose. Don't worry about whether swimming burns more calories than cycling—the bottom line is that any activity that gets you moving and off the couch will burn calories and help you on your way to living a Skinny life.

Why do you have to love it? Because, let's face it, if you hate to run and you set a goal of running for 30 minutes every day, how likely is it that you'll actually meet that goal?

Maybe it would happen for a few days or even a few weeks, but you'll be fighting an uphill battle to do it consistently. Most of all, loving what you do will help you to be consistent with exercise—a Skinny rule for any workout plan.

Changing your exercise routine can help you continue to love working out, too! Try a new workout DVD, pick a new walking route, join a yoga class, work out with a personal trainer, bike, kayak, ski, play a sport, shoot hoops. Create the perfect combination of what is right for you and it will help you to love exercise and the Skinny self that comes along with it! 🆂🆁

Three

Skinny Foods

SKINNY
RULE
36

Think about
What You *Must* Eat

Most times when people think about losing weight, they think about what foods to cut out. Yet Skinny people do just the opposite: They think about what foods to add in! Adding the right type of foods to your diet will help to keep you feeling full and satisfied rather than always wanting more. Nutrition expert David Grotto, RD, LDN, explains in his book *101 Optimal Foods,* "The most important tip that changed my entire practice is to focus on only using an add-in approach." Grotto notes that focusing on what foods to take away just doesn't work as effectively as working more on what foods you can add in.

Eat More 'Errys

Some specific favorite foods Grotto recommends that his clients add are any foods ending in *erry!* Meaning: blue-b*erry,* cranb*erry,* strawb*erry,* blackb*erry.* These foods are all loaded with antioxidants and anthocyanins, which have been linked to improved vascular flexibility.

Eat More Whole Grains

Another food that I suggest folks add in is whole grains, like whole-wheat bread, brown rice, whole-grain cous-cous, old-fashioned rolled oats and whole-wheat pasta. Making the swap from "regular" white versions of grain foods will help keep your belly full because of the fiber. Plus, as an added health benefit, whole grains have more of what I like to call "behind the scenes" nutrients, like selenium, potassium and magnesium.

Don't fall for look-alike grains (foods that look like they are whole grain but are really just colored with caramel coloring and are not truly 100 percent whole grain). When you are grocery shopping, look for grains that say on the packaging "100% whole wheat," have whole wheat as the first ingredient on the list and have at least three grams of dietary fiber per serving.

Here is a great Skinny recipe to have at breakfast to add more whole grains to your diet:

Skinny Oatmeal

Serves 1

Ingredients

1 cup cooked rolled oats (not instant)

1 tablespoon chopped walnuts

1/4 cup dried cranberries

Directions

Cook oatmeal according to package directions (1/2 cup dry oatmeal will yield 1 cup cooked oatmeal). Then mix in nuts and dried fruit. YUM!

Nutrition Facts (per serving)

300 calories, 8 grams fat, 1 gram saturated fat, 0 grams trans fat, 0 mg cholesterol, 0 mg sodium, 53 grams carbohydrates, 6 grams fiber, 21 grams sugar, 7 grams protein

Drink More Black and Green Teas

Grotto also recommends that people drink more black and green teas. These teas provide flavonoids and caffeine that studies have shown lead to decreased dementia and improved cognitive function. A favorite drink of mine is an "Arnold Palmer," named after the golf legend and known for its refreshing taste. Here is my Skinny version of the traditional drink. It's simple and still very tasty!

Skinny Arnold Palmer

Serves 1

Ingredients

1 green tea bag

16 ounces hot water

1 teaspoon lemon juice

1 teaspoon sugar

Directions

1. In a tall glass, add water and then let the tea bag steep for about 3 to 5 minutes.

2. Stir in lemon juice and sugar!

This drink only has about 15 calories per glass and 4 grams of sugar, compared to the 28 grams of sugar in a 16-ounce glass of store-bought Arnold Palmer Iced Tea Lemonade.

Nutrition Facts (per 16 ounces)

15 calories, 0 grams fat, 0 grams saturated fat, 0 grams trans fat, 0 mg cholesterol, 0 mg sodium, 4 grams carbohydrates, 0 grams fiber, 4 grams sugar, 0 grams protein

Eat More Garlic, Apples and Iron for Energy and Performance

When it comes to boosting physical performance, Grotto suggests a few specific foods: garlic, apples and iron-rich foods. Garlic is known to have a fatigue-fighting impact on the body, thanks to its powerful phytochemical profile, including allicin, saponin and coumaric acid. "An apple a day gets you to move out of the way," states Grotto, due to the polyphenols that are linked to improved physical and athletic performance. A trend Grotto has noticed is that people tend to have underlying anemia, which can result in fatigue; adding in foods that provide iron will help to curb the problem. Among iron-rich foods are shrimp, beans, potatoes with skin, prunes (dried plums), pumpkin seeds and, of course, red meat. Combine those foods with a small glass of orange juice, some red bell pepper or another food that is rich in vitamin C to enhance the absorption of the iron by the body.

Use this Skinny rule to help motivate you to start thinking a little differently about food by placing more of a focus on what foods to add in rather than what foods to take away. ⑤

| SKINNY RULE **37** | **Eat Fewer Processed Foods** |

Just as Skinny girls eat more good-for-them foods, they also focus on eating more foods that are less processed. Take this nutrition tip from Marisa Miller, who was featured in the 2008 *Sports Illustrated* swimsuit issue: "My main thing is not eating processed food," says the model. What does this mean? Eating foods in their most natural forms without the added preservatives, fillers and other additives. Instead, stick to whole foods like fruits, vegetables, lean meats, whole-grain breads and low-fat dairy foods.

Skinny people accomplish this by shopping the perimeter of the grocery store first, which is where you will find these whole foods and ensure that your cart is filling up with the right stuff. In the middle of the grocery store are processed foods, which are all foods you want to eliminate or limit in your diet.

Here is the skinny on what foods to pile in your cart: In the produce section, put in your cart a variety of fruits and vegetables. Challenge yourself each shopping trip to try a new or unusual fruit or veggie and then learn how to prepare it. Here are a few to try: leeks, rutabaga, parsnips, pomegranates, kumquats and star fruit. Don't forget to stock up on fresh herbs, like rosemary, cilantro and parsley. When it comes to bread, try to pick up whole-wheat bread products from the in-store bakery; these products have fewer additives than many of the prepackaged bread options.

As Michael Pollan urges in his book, *In Defense of Food,* aim to eat real, unprocessed food. When you are sifting through the thousands of bags, boxes and cans of food, try this Skinny tip: Before reading the Nutrition Facts panel, read the ingredient list. If there are any words you can't pronounce, put it back. If there are more than five or so ingredients, put it back. This simple trick will get you well on your way to eating fewer processed foods.

A fun challenge to try is to make a meal just from the perimeter of the store! Think about it: You really don't need to grab foods from the center aisles. For example: grilled salmon, served over sautéed spinach (okay, head into the center aisles for extra virgin olive oil) and a baked sweet potato. A perfectly balanced, tasty and unprocessed dinner— all from the perimeter of the grocery store! **SR**

Skinny Tip

Simply going grocery shopping is a Skinny little secret. Why? Most important, it will keep your fruit bowl stocked and your refrigerator full of fresh foods. Also, grocery shopping for 30 minutes burns about 100 calories. So next time you're thinking of ordering takeout instead of getting groceries and cooking, remember this Skinny secret and go grocery shopping instead.

SKINNY RULE 38

Choose Foods with Color

Here's a Skinny secret that you may have heard before, but it's so important it's worth repeating: Pile your plate with lots of color in order to get a range of essential vitamins and nutrients from your food. All colors of the spectrum in some shape or form contribute health benefits, from white to deep, dark purple! Dr. Andrew Weil explains on his website, www.drweil.com, that the vibrant colors of fruits and vegetables may, in fact, be nature's way of attracting us to them.

So what exactly do all the colors have to offer? Reds, like tomatoes, strawberries and watermelon, have lycopene, which is a powerful antioxidant that has been known to fight heart disease and certain types of cancer. Orange and yellow fruits and vegetables, like carrots, mangoes, yellow bell peppers and cantaloupe, provide the body with beta-carotene, a known immune-system booster. Green foods, like spinach, broccoli, romaine and kiwi, contain antioxidants like lutein and zeaxanthin that have been linked to helping eyesight. The blues and purples, found in foods like blueberries, red cabbage, beets, plums and purple grapes, are loaded with the phytochemical anthocyanin, which may help to prevent heart disease. White foods, like onions and garlic, provide allicin that has been linked to reducing cholesterol and blood pressure.

By adding a variety of colors to your eating routine you will be reaping the health benefits coming from the entire rainbow of foods. Here are a few tasty, Skinny and easy recipes to brighten your eating routine with a variety of colors.

Skinny Spinach

Serves 4
Includes red, orange, yellow, green and white

Ingredients

1 bag fresh baby spinach

1 clove garlic, minced

½ red bell pepper, chopped

½ orange pepper, chopped

½ yellow pepper, chopped

Extra virgin olive oil

Directions

1. In a sauté pan, drizzle a small amount (less than a teaspoon) of extra virgin olive oil and start sautéing the chopped peppers.

2. Once the peppers are tender, add the minced garlic and spinach. Sauté for about 2 minutes until the spinach is wilted.

Nutrition Facts (per serving)

40 calories, 1 gram fat, 0 grams saturated fat, 0 grams trans fat, 0 mg cholesterol, 60 mg sodium, 7 grams carbohydrates, 3 grams fiber, 2 grams sugar, 3 grams protein

Skinny Fruit Kabobs

Serves 4
Includes red, orange, green and blue/purple

Ingredients

8 medium wooden skewers

½ cup watermelon, cubed into bite-size pieces

½ cup cantaloupe, cubed into bite-size pieces

½ cup mango, chopped into bite-size pieces

2 kiwi, chopped

½ cup red grapes

½ cup blackberries

Directions

1. Randomly place the rainbow of fruit on skewers.

2. Chill and enjoy!

Nutrition Facts (per serving)

60 calories, 0 grams fat, 0 grams saturated fat, 0 grams trans fat, 0 mg cholesterol, 5 mg sodium, 14 grams carbohydrates, 3 grams fiber, 10 grams sugar, 1 gram protein 🆂🅁

SKINNY RULE 39 — Clean Your Cupboards

Skinny people don't have overstuffed pantries and cupboards. Although it may be tempting to stock up on foods when they are on sale and have cupboards full of different options, you're not helping yourself by doing so. Follow this Skinny rule and limit the number of foods you have on hand instead.

Keeping your cupboards nice and clean will help you become more focused when choosing foods at the grocery store and limit the number of temptations available when you get the munchies. This holds true even for healthier foods, like nuts and whole-grain crackers. While they provide your body with great nutrients, they still come with a heavy calorie price tag. The bottom line to getting and keeping your weight down is limiting the number of calories you consume every day.

Calorie price tag example: A serving of almonds (1 ounce) has 165 calories.

Calorie deal to stock up on: Air-popped popcorn (make it yourself); 1 cup has 31 calories.

Less processed foods to keep on hand so you can whip together a nutritionally balanced meal in minutes to keep snacking in check:

- Beans: black beans, chickpeas, pinto beans
- Brown rice
- Quinoa
- Whole-wheat pasta

Strive to keep less processed foods in your cupboards or pantries. As an added bonus, by cutting down on the boxes in your cupboards, you cut down on processed foods—an essential Skinny rule! 🆂🆁

SKINNY RULE 40

Try These Belly-Blasting Foods

While your primary motivation to get rid of belly fat may be more about how your jeans fit, there's another goal you can keep in mind for motivation: That extra fat around the middle puts you at risk for heart disease and type 2 diabetes.

More and more research continues to come out about what types of food will blast away belly fat. This is very exciting because, for the longest time, nutrition experts said that there wasn't a connection between the types of food we ate and body fat in specific regions of the body. That made trimming weight around the middle that much more daunting. Belly fat is visceral body fat, a type of fat that lies deep down inside your midsection and surrounds major organs, including the heart and liver.

Research done by the Yale-Griffin Prevention Research Center on the study of *Prevention*'s *Flat Belly Diet!,* co-created by *Prevention*'s editor-in-chief, Liz Vaccariello, showed that following a diet rich in monounsaturated fats decreased visceral belly fat by as much as 33 percent!

The overarching, common thread among all the research is that foods rich in monounsaturated fats (MUFAs) have been proven to decrease body fat, especially the dreaded fat around the middle. There are many foods that provide belly-blasting amounts of MUFA. Try working these foods into your eating routine: avocado, extra virgin olive oil, almonds, sunflower seeds, pumpkin seeds and peanut butter.

Another study, published in the *American Journal of Clinical Nutrition,* found that adults eating whole grains during a 12-week program lost double the fat in the belly area as compared to the group who ate refined grains (aka white-grain products). The study concludes that because whole grains contain more fiber, which naturally slows digestion and prevents blood sugar levels from spiking too quickly, this results in lower insulin levels. Moreover, lower insulin levels seem to be linked to decreased fat-cell sizes in the midsection. Foods to include in your eating routine that are good sources of whole grains are whole-wheat cereal, oatmeal, brown rice, barley, whole-grain bread and whole-wheat pasta.

Here are suggestions about how to incorporate monounsaturated fats and whole grains in your diet to say good-bye to belly fat.

AT BREAKFAST: Choose whole-wheat cereals, whole-wheat toast with a light spread of peanut butter or try oatmeal with a handful of berries and walnuts.

FOR SNACKS: Try whole-wheat crackers with hummus, a small handful of nuts and an apple or a slice of whole-wheat bread with almond butter.

AT LUNCH: Add a small handful of olives and nuts on your salad. Instead of salad dressing, choose a drizzle of balsamic vinegar and extra virgin olive oil. Opt for whole-wheat pasta with sauce and grilled chicken.

FOR DINNER: Serve side dishes like barley, brown rice and beans, whole-wheat pasta tossed with extra virgin olive oil, a handful of olives and a dash of Parmesan cheese.

Lastly, grab this recipe for Sassy Water from the *Flat Belly Diet!,* and keep a pitcher of this on hand in the refrigerator to further decrease belly bloating. Here's the recipe:

Sassy Water

Ingredients

2 liters water (about 8½ cups)

1 teaspoon freshly grated ginger

1 medium cucumber, peeled and thinly sliced

1 medium lemon, thinly sliced

12 small spearmint leaves

Directions

Combine all the ingredients in a large pitcher and let the flavors blend overnight. Drink the entire pitcher by the end of each day. ⑤⑫

SKINNY
RULE
41

Snack throughout the Day

E ating throughout the day is a Skinny must. Try eating about every three to four hours with light meals and mini meals for snacks. A Skinny and satisfying eating schedule might look like this:

> 8:00 a.m. Breakfast
> 10:30 a.m. Light Snack
> 1:00 p.m. Lunch
> 4:00 p.m. Light Snack
> 7:30 p.m. Dinner

Research published in the *American Journal of Epidemiology* took a look at the eating patterns of 499 people. The study found that eating frequently throughout the day was associated with a lower risk of obesity. Eating frequently was defined as four or more eating "episodes" a day, as opposed to three or fewer.

Think about your day and how frequently your eating episodes are. If you are a meal skipper, use this tip as motivation to revamp your eating patterns and step up the number of your eating episodes. It will help you shave pounds and satisfy your appetite!

About 15 minutes before a meal, grab an apple (or another fiber-packed fruit, like a handful of raspberries). Research by Penn State has showed that the simple act of eating an apple (calorie cost: about 128 calories) 15 minutes before a meal left the study participants feeling full and more satisfied after their meal and resulted in eating 187 fewer calories during the meal. The net savings of about 60 calories may seem minimal, but a daily savings of 60 calories results in a savings of 420 calories per week and a Skinny savings of 21,840 calories over the course of the year—pounds worth of calories saved!

Skinny Tip

But rather than haphazardly choosing the food from your fridge for your meals and snacks, balance each snack and meal with a blend of carbohydrates, protein and fats. This will help you feel more satisfied than snacking on salty or sugary treats and goodies. Some Skinny snack ideas: fresh berries with plain yogurt and a drizzle of honey; celery sticks with a light spread of peanut butter; a handful of almonds and dried fruit; a cup of low-fat, pineapple-flavored cottage cheese; or a few whole-grain crackers dipped in roasted red pepper hummus (a favorite of mine). ⑤

SKINNY
RULE
42

Balance Energy Intake

D id you know that calories are actually a unit of energy? Every pound of weight is equal to 3,500 calories. So if you want to lose 10 pounds, that means through food choices and exercise you have to find a way to cut out and/or burn up 35,000 calories. That is a lot of energy, right? It is important to know the math of gaining and losing weight because it helps put calories in a different perspective. Being Skinny is all about balancing energy (calories) in versus energy (calories) out. Skinny people know little ways to save calories here and there. While it may be just a few calories of savings, every calorie counts! Here is a quick lesson about weight and balancing calories.

Check out this example: One little piece of M&M candy has about 3 calories. Say you grab a handful of these tasty little treats and scoop up 10 pieces—you've just consumed 30 calories. Now figure that you do this two times a day. That will add up to a total of 60 calories per day. Then, say you do this every day for a year—that adds up to a whopping 21,900 calories, or about six pounds' worth of calories over the course of a year. Of course, this does not mean that you should avoid eating M&Ms altogether, but you need to know how much every little calorie impacts your bottom line. In fact, if you love M&Ms, a Skinny rule would be to give in to your craving for the little chocolate treats, control the portion and account for the calories.

Even dipping into the hard candy dish can push the energy balance equation out of balance in a hurry! Each hard candy has about five calories. Five seemingly harmless candies per day over the course of a year will add up to about five pounds' worth of calories.

Keep this Skinny calorie equation in mind the next time you are tempted by the shiny little packaged candies at the bank, at the office, on your coworker's desk, on your grandma's coffee table or just about anywhere else you turn.

Take a moment to think of all the ways extra calories are slipping into your routine and start by making a strategy to eliminate them. Note that *extra* is the key word here, meaning you should focus on looking for sources of unnecessary calories. This differentiation is important because if you eliminate calories that are providing healthful nutrients like those from fruit, you are also cutting out all the health benefits that come along with those calories. Rather, if you work on cutting out added fats and sugar, you won't wind up skimping on foods that are abundant in nutrients.

So, are you adding sugar to your coffee every morning? Grabbing goodies from a candy dish? Spreading butter on your bread? Remember, every calorie eliminated makes a difference in the overall calorie balance equation. Challenge yourself to cut out unnecessary calories to reach your Skinny goals.

On a similar note, every time you burn up a few more calories, you're moving the calorie balance equation in the right direction! See Part Two: Skinny Fitness for more on exercise and burning up calories. ⊛

<table>
<tr><td>SKINNY
RULE
43</td><td># Fill the Fruit Bowl</td></tr>
</table>

Okay, you may be thinking, what is the big deal about filling the fruit bowl? Although this may seem and maybe is one of the easiest tips in the book, it is one of the most essential Skinny rules to follow! When I help my clients figure out ways to improve their eating habits, we always discuss how they can add more fruit to their diet. And I'm always shocked to hear the reason why most of my clients aren't getting in their daily fill of fruit: They don't keep it in the house. It's practically impossible to eat more fruits without having them on hand, so although this seems like something that is fairly simple and obvious, keeping a full fruit bowl is a definite Skinny must.

Keep some staples, like apples and bananas, on hand in a fruit bowl all the time. Then in the crisper drawer of your refrigerator, keep a stash of your favorites. Some of my favorites are oranges and mangoes.

Another Skinny tip! When you buy fruit that needs preparation, do it right when you get home from the store. Wash the fruit, cut it, prepare it and place it in airtight containers. Then it is ready to go when you are hungry for it and when you open the refrigerator wondering what there is to eat, you'll see ready-to-go containers of fruit that will make it easy to grab and go.

To inspire you to pick up the fruit over the other goodies in the fridge, try keeping the fruit out of your crisper drawer, up on a shelf where it will be at eye level. Okay, I know I just told you to keep the crisper drawer full, but this portion of the Skinny rule is for all of you who routinely find pieces of fruit growing fur in the crisper drawer.

This rule expands beyond the fruit bowl and applies to the refrigerator and cupboards, too. Keeping a kitchen and pantry stocked with Skinny foods is a key to living the Skinny life. 🆂🆁

| SKINNY RULE **44** | Try These Top 10 Lowest-Calorie Veggies |

Veggies are a Skinny girl's best friend because they pack important nutrients with few calories. In fact, if you know people who go to Weight Watchers, they will likely be quick to tell you how vegetables are considered "free" foods! I actually like to encourage people to think of vegetables as "full" foods because vegetables are full of health-promoting nutrients and belly-filling fiber. Choosing vegetables (this goes for fruit, too) in a variety of colors is a great way to vary the nutrients that your body is getting.

Try to sneak these 10 Skinniest, lowest-calorie vegetables into your diet on a regular basis:

Vegetable	Serving Size	Calories
Spinach	1 cup	7
Romaine Lettuce	1 cup	10
Radish Slices	1 cup	19
Diced Celery	1 cup	19
Summer Squash	1 cup	20
Asparagus	1 cup	27

continued

Vegetable	Serving Size	Calories
Snap Peas	1 cup	34
Green Beans	1 cup	34
Chopped Tomatoes	1 cup	38
Chopped Carrots	1 cup	52

While we're talking about some of the vegetables with the lowest calorie content, it's important to talk about the vegetables that get a bad rap—the starchy vegetables like potatoes. Despite their un-Skinny reputation, one cup of boiled potatoes has only 130 calories and about 3 grams of fiber! In the grand scheme of calorie balance, 130 calories from starchy vegetables is much better than 130 calories from snack foods or cookies that don't have the vitamins, nutrients and fiber that potatoes do.

A good rule of thumb to follow when selecting vegetables is to choose the Skinnier vegetables, like those listed above, more often and the starchy vegetables less often. But there is no reason for you to skip the starchy veggies altogether! In fact, they are a great way to add variety to your eating routine while keeping your taste buds piqued and still providing your body with important nutrients and fiber.

Just as with fruit, it is important to choose a variety of vegetables in all different colors. Be adventurous and introduce new veggies into your diet. Some less well-known vegetables to try: bok choy, leeks, beets, parsnips, edamame (aka soybeans), scallions (aka green onions) and shallots. Each of these offer great flavor with a low-calorie, Skinny price tag.

Just as with fruit, when you buy veggies, thoroughly wash and slice up your cucumbers, tomatoes and carrots as soon as you get home from the store and place them in airtight storage containers or bags. That way, you'll be able to grab them on short notice. Even consider which veggies you may pack in a lunch or take with you as a snack on the go. For example, while you are slicing cucumbers, make a few single-serving containers or bags, so even when you're in a hurry you have tasty Skinny foods ready to go. Another fun Skinny tip is to take a clear storage container that fits on the top shelf of your refrigerator and place your single-serving containers or bags of ready-to-go veggies (and fruit) in it. Keeping them at eye level will remind you that they are there! 🅢🅡

| SKINNY RULE 45 | Read Ingredient Lists—and Know What to Avoid |

Picking up a food package and trying to read the ingredient list can be a surprisingly difficult task. Oftentimes, the ingredient list contains words and ingredients you don't even recognize! That is kind of scary when you consider that you have no idea what the heck butylated hydroxyanisole (BHA) is, but you are going to put it in your body nonetheless. You may be thinking, What is this? Is this healthy? Or isn't it healthy? The Center for Science in the Public Interest defines BHA as an ingredient that slows rancidity in fats, oils and fat-containing foods, and while some studies show that it is safe, others show that it causes cancer in rats, mice and hamsters. In fact, the U.S. Department of Health and Human Services reports that BHA is "reasonably anticipated to be a human carcinogen."

The simplest way to deal with this dilemma when selecting foods is to keep it simple and look for those with the fewest ingredients on the list. Better yet, try to challenge yourself to incorporate more foods that don't even have ingredient lists, like fruits, vegetables and natural meat and dairy products. This is an essential Skinny rule and it lessens the need to translate the seemingly hard-to-understand world of food technology.

So what do those big words really mean and which ones should you avoid? Partially hydrogenated oil is an ingredient to avoid. If a food includes partially hydrogenated oil on the ingredient list, this means that the product has trans fats in it, which is a type of fat that is particularly bad for your heart. Trans fats have been all over the news lately because of how unhealthy they are; in response, many food manufacturers have scrambled to reformulate food products so the packaging can tout "0 grams of trans fat." Yet, those very foods can actually still have trans fat in them. How is that so? Because food-labeling regulations allow manufacturers to list 0 grams of trans fat (this applies to total and saturated fat, too) when there is up to 0.4 grams of trans fat per serving. Yes, this means that a product that boasts 0 grams of trans fat can actually have trans fat in it. So keep it Skinny by avoiding foods with *partially hydrogenated oil* in the ingredient list at all.

AVOID THESE!

Ingredients to avoid, according to the Center for Science in the Public Interest (CSPI):

Acesulfame Potassium

Artificial Colorings: Blue 2, Green 3, Orange B, Red 3, Yellow 5, Yellow 6

Aspartame

Butylated Hydroxyanisole

Hydrogenated Oil

Partially Hydrogenated Oil

Potassium Bromate

Propyl Gallate

Saccharin

Sodium Nitrate

Sodium Nitrite

In addition to avoiding certain ingredients, one ingredient to make sure is at the very top of your list when choosing cereal, breads and pasta should be whole wheat! The reason? Many grain products are made to look like they are whole grain because they are brown in color, but in fact they may not really be whole wheat. The words *enriched grains* sounds fancy, as if it may be a good thing. Yet what it means is that your bread is made with grains that have been stripped of their nutrients and then they have had the mandated nutrients added back in. Keep in mind that even though some nutrients are added back in, the nutrients found in the whole grain (like fiber) are still missing. ⬤

SKINNY RULE **46**	Shop for Groceries the Skinny Way—without Breaking the Bank

Just as there's a Skinny and an un-Skinny way to eat, there's a Skinny and an un-Skinny way to grocery-shop. To shop like a Skinny girl, stick to the perimeter of the grocery store. Stop and think about this for a minute: The perimeter is where you traditionally find wholesome foods, like fresh fruit and vegetables, meats, milk and dairy, breads, eggs and so on—all foods that should be a regular part of your Skinny diet. What's in those center aisles? Processed foods, loaded with sugars, additives and trans fats—not Skinny at all!

Even go so far as to shop the perimeter of the grocery store first, filling up your cart with the good stuff and leaving less room for the processed foods that are found in the center of the store. Now you may be thinking, Are those foods going to cost more and drive up my grocery bill? Sadly enough, yes. Whole foods do cost more. Yet, interestingly, food costs less today than it did in 1966. *Time* magazine reports in a recent article titled "Getting Real About the High Price of Cheap Food," that according to the USDA, Americans spend less than 10 percent of their incomes on food, down from 18 percent in 1966. The article also highlights findings from a study in the *American Journal of Clinical Nutrition* that found that $1 could buy 1,200 calories of potato chips or 875 calories of soda but just 250 calories of vegetables or 170 calories of fresh fruit.

How to save calories and money? Try these Skinny saving tips to shop the perimeter of the grocery store without breaking the bank. In the produce section, choose fruit and vegetables that are in season because they tend to cost less. And, whenever possible, go to a local farm stand instead of the grocery store. Always keep bananas on hand because they typically cost only 20 cents each or less. Look for economy-size bags of produce, like sweet potatoes, carrots, onions and apples. You can typically save on the per pound price when buying a larger quantity and, as an added bonus, when you have more fruits and veggies readily available in the fridge, you will wind up eating more of them, too!

When you are shopping for meats, look for value packs. Cooking for one or two? Then when you get home, split up the value pack into smaller portions, place them in freezer bags and freeze them to use at a later date. In the meat, poultry and seafood sections, stick to the leanest cuts available. For example: 95 percent lean ground beef, filet mignon, center-cut pork chops, pork tenderloin, chicken tenders, boneless, skinless chicken breasts. In the seafood aisle, try to add to your cart heart-healthy fish on a weekly basis, like salmon, mackerel and albacore tuna.

In the dairy section of the grocery store, look for low-fat or 1 percent or less milk and other dairy products for the Skinniest options. Great items to pick up: light sour cream, low-fat cottage cheese, 1 percent or low-fat milk and low-fat or fat-free yogurt. Always buy low-fat or skim milk by the gallon. While the price of milk varies from time to time, one cup of milk, when purchased in a gallon-size container costs only about 22 cents per serving. The good thing is that one gallon of milk should only last a few days, considering that you should be striving to have three one-cup servings of milk or other dairy foods per day (see Skinny Rule #49, Get Your Three Every Day).

Another key to Skinny grocery shopping is shopping with a list—check out Skinny Rule #50, Make a List and Check It Twice, for more on this. ⑤

SKINNY
RULE
47

Don't Judge a Food by Its Package

T his one Skinny rule could be expanded into an entire book! Food packages these days look like racecars with all the symbols and advertising on them to try and make them seem healthy. Even worse, most of the "healthy" symbols you see on food packaging were developed by the food manufacturers themselves. The Skinny rule: Don't fall for good-for-you labels; use your own sound judgment when making food choices.

A perfect example of false packaging is one of the newest labeling symbol systems, called the Smart Choices Program™. The Smart Choices Program is backed by the nation's largest food manufacturers, who pay up to $100,000 a year to be part of the program, with a fee based on total sales of the products that show the seal. The seal is a green checkmark label that will be showing up on the front of hundreds of food packages, including sugary items like Froot Loops and Apple Jacks that aren't good for you by any means. As Walter C. Willet, chairman of the Nutrition Department at the Harvard School of Public Health told the *New York Times,* "These are horrible choices." He goes on to note that the criteria used by the Smart Choices Program are seriously flawed, allowing less healthy products, like sugary cereals, to win its seal of approval.

The good news is that there are independent systems coming out now to rate foods and highlight those that are truly nutritionally balanced. One example of an independent system is NuVal, which was started by Dr. David Katz and a team funded by Griffin Hospital, a nonprofit community and teaching hospital affiliated with the Yale University School of Medicine. This system uses a science-based algorithm to rate foods from every section of the grocery store on a scale of 1 to 100. The higher the score, the higher the nutrient density. While the scoring is complex, the bottom line is that only the healthiest foods throughout the grocery store get top scores, like skim milk, wheat bran, shredded wheat, blueberries and spinach. Processed foods get scored as well, but they have much lower scores. This system is currently being used by several grocery stores and will likely continue to grow in popularity due to its grounding in sound science.

So what does this all mean to you? When you grocery-shop, there are going to be tons of different systems, stamps and seals glaring at you, trying to convince you that a food is healthy! Follow your Skinny instincts and let your common sense rise above all that fancy packaging. Ultimately, remember that you are the gatekeeper of what foods do and do not end up in your grocery cart and in your kitchen. Even more important, most of the confusion arises in the middle aisles of the grocery store where a majority of the processed foods are kept. Even more reason to follow Skinny Rule #46 and shop for groceries the Skinny way. Do most of your shopping along the perimeter of the grocery store and you will primarily be choosing wholesome, healthier foods, like whole-grain breads, fruit, vegetables, milk and lean meats—no fancy packaging needed! ⑤⑧

| SKINNY RULE **48** | Snack Like a Skinny Girl |

A s you know from Skinny Rule #41, the perfect Skinny diet includes breakfast, a light snack, lunch, a light snack and dinner. Notice the word *light* before every snack—that word is key to snacking the Skinny way. Portion size is just as, if not more, important than choosing Skinny snacks.

The trick to making this schedule work for you is to snack the Skinny way—choose balanced snacks (with healthy carbs, protein and fats) and watch your portions. And if you're craving something in particular? Giving into your cravings is truly a Skinny solution (see Skinny Rules #14 and #16) with one important caveat: portion control. Say, you're like me and you love ice cream. Giving in to your craving doesn't mean you have a green light to indulge in a five-scoop sundae, loaded with toppings and piled high with whipped cream. Sorry! In the case of ice cream, what it does mean is enjoying a serving of ice cream, which I am sad to announce is only ½ cup or the size of half a baseball, and enjoying every bite of it.

While giving in to your cravings occasionally, don't fall into the trap of making all your snacks sweets, because even if you keep the portion size in check, they are lacking important nutrients and health-promoting antioxidants.

Instead, some fantastic Skinny snack solutions include the following:

- 3 cups of air-popped (or plain) popcorn
- 1 cup of berries with a small dollop of whipped cream
- an apple and a part-skim mozzarella cheese stick
- 1 cup of low-fat milk and a graham cracker
- a small handful of dried fruit and walnuts
- 1 cup of low-fat, plain yogurt topped with fruit
- a smoothie made with plain, low-fat yogurt and frozen fruit

Or you can take a cue from some Skinny celebs, who shared their go-to snacks with www.self.com: Andrea Roth and Callie Thorne of *Rescue Me* snack on fresh fruit; Kellee Stewart of *My Boys* loves tuna salad (made with low-fat mayo, capers and scallions) with wheat thins; and Michaela Conlin of *Bones* chooses unsalted raw cashews.

As for my favorite Skinny snacks: air-popped popcorn, pineapple and cottage cheese, a cup of fresh mango, a small handful of dried cranberries and cashews or an orange. All have just the right amount of sweetness to tide me over and they even feel like a treat!

A word of caution on snacking at night: While planning a night snack can be a great idea and can help you get a good night's rest, this can be a time of day when people overdo it, indulging in large portions because they're relaxed and may be sitting and eating mindlessly at the computer or in front of the television. That said, if you find yourself overdoing it at night, even if you are eating so-called healthy foods, here are a few Skinny solutions to try. One would be to skip the night snack altogether. Second, try to portion out your snack onto a plate after dinner and leave it in the cupboard for your snacktime. Third, brush your teeth immediately after your snack to keep you from grabbing seconds or thirds. How you cope with nighttime snacking really depends on you. Some people start snacking at night, and seem to graze all night before bed. This is a habit that you've gotta break. A better option would be to drink a cup of low-fat, warmed milk or a cup of herbal tea, like chamomile, which have a soothing effect. 𝕊𝕣

SKINNY RULE 49

Get Your Three Every Day

Usually, when you read headlines that say things like SIMPLE WAY TO LOSE WEIGHT, MIRACLE CURE FOR WEIGHT LOSS and other outrageous claims, you know they are too good to be true. But this is the exception to the rule. New research shows that having three servings of low-fat dairy foods per day promotes a healthy weight and specifically helps to decrease belly fat!

While scientists are not 100 percent sure why dairy foods promote weight loss, one possible explanation is that the nutrients in dairy foods help the body run more efficiently, promoting weight loss when coupled with a balanced, low-calorie eating plan. For example, take calcium, a key nutrient in dairy. Ninety-nine percent of calcium is stored in bones and teeth and the remaining 1 percent aids in muscle contraction, nerve function and hormone production. Calcium is just one of the nine essential nutrients that dairy foods provide. The other eight are potassium, phosphorus, magnesium, vitamin A, vitamin D, riboflavin, protein and vitamin B12. Given all the nutrients dairy foods provide, you could say milk is the original energy drink!

You may have noticed the words above—*low-calorie eating plan*. It's important to factor those three servings of dairy a day into your total calorie goals to promote a healthy weight.

So what does three servings per day really look like? One serving of low-fat dairy foods would be: 1 cup of milk, 1 cup of yogurt, 1 ounce of cheese. And watch out for big glasses—one cup literally means eight ounces, no matter what the size of the glass. And be sure to choose low-fat dairy foods—they provide the very same nine essential nutrients with fewer calories and less fat. When you are purchasing dairy foods, look for the following: Fat-free (0%) or Low-fat (1%).

A perfect solution for getting the recommended three servings of low-fat dairy foods every day is to have a serving at breakfast, lunch and dinner. Try this Skinny combination: 1 cup of yogurt at breakfast, 1 ounce part-skim mozzarella cheese at lunch and 1 cup of milk at dinner. ⑤⑧

SKINNY RULE 50
Make a List and Check It Twice

If you've ever left the grocery store without something you need, read this Skinny rule very carefully and use it on your very next grocery shopping trip. Think of your grocery list as your plan of attack. After all, the grocery store is set up with products strategically arranged to entice you to buy them. It's really a jungle in there, and without a plan of attack you will easily get lost, waste money and most likely leave without something you wanted to get in the first place!

Ideally, the first step in making your grocery list is creating your meal plan for the week. Plan at least a week's worth of meals. This doesn't have to be a time-intensive exercise—it can be done quite quickly—and the more you do it, the easier it becomes. To get started, ask yourself: What do I want to have for breakfast this week? How many days do I need to pack a lunch (take into account any work meetings or lunch plans you have)? How many nights do I need to cook dinner? What foods do I need to keep on hand to make healthy snacks easily accessible? What is going to be the one snack/treat I purchase for the week?

Once you have thought through these questions, you can start planning. Ideally, plan one or two different breakfasts for the week. For example, a smoothie for three days and whole-wheat toast with peanut butter for the remaining four days. With lunch, if you're planning to make your own lunch for four days, try something like salads for two of the days and wraps for two of the days. If you're going to eat dinner at home five nights, try cooking three of those nights and enjoying leftovers on the other two nights. For snacks, you can pick up popping corn to air-pop, fresh fruit or low-fat yogurt. For the treat, grab one bag, box or container (and not the jumbo size!) of your favorite snack food.

Now start making your list of what you need, based on your plan. Once you have made your list, it's time to do the crucial next step and check it twice: Cross-reference your shopping list with what is already in your kitchen, and cross off the items on your list that you already have.

This last component takes just an extra quick minute and is totally worth it. Organize your list by how you walk through the grocery store. If you walk into produce first, have fruits and vegetables at the top of your list. Next you head to the seafood and meat counter, so place those items on your list next and so on. This Skinny organizational strategy will help you stay on task and focused during your next grocery shopping trip. It may also save you money by keeping you from overbuying foods that you don't need. ⑤⑫

SKINNY RULE

51

Put the Power of Portions to Work for You

A Skinny insider secret is to eat and enjoy any food, but watch the portion. By watching the portion I don't mean watching three huge heaping scoops of ice cream go into your dish—it means keeping the portion size of any and all foods in check.

Registered dietitian Lisa Young, PhD, RD, author of *The Portion Teller,* puts this well when she explains, "People should be more concerned about *how* much they are eating, rather than getting wrapped up with *what* they are eating."

Paying close attention to portion size makes a huge difference in any eating plan because the calorie balance equation is a very delicate one. And overeating, even on healthy foods like sweet potatoes, almonds and peanut butter, can lead to weight gain. However, most would agree that where people get in trouble is by consuming oversized portions of less healthy foods like potato chips, cookies and ice cream, as these foods pile on calories much more quickly than many healthier options.

Young has some great practical ways to rein in the portions of all foods. Check them out:

Nonstarchy Vegetables (e.g., carrots, tomatoes)

1 cup raw = 1 baseball
½ cup cooked = ½ baseball

Fruit (e.g., apple, grapes, peach, dried fruit, pear)

1 medium apple, 1 cup grapes, 1 peach = 1 baseball
¼ cup dried fruit = 1 golf ball
1 pear = 1 lightbulb

Starchy Vegetables (e.g., corn, potatoes)

½ cup cooked corn = ½ baseball
½ cup boiled potatoes = ½ baseball
3-4-ounce baked potato with skin = ½ computer mouse

Whole Grains (e.g., oatmeal, brown rice, pancake)

⅔ cup cooked oatmeal = 1 tennis ball
½ cup cooked brown rice = ½ baseball
1-ounce pancake = diameter of CD

Meat, Fish, Poultry

3-4 ounces cooked meat, fish or poultry = 1 deck of cards

If you are unsure of your portion size, start using Lisa Young's visualizing techniques or even break out the measuring cups. Actually scoop one serving of cereal into your bowl (check the serving size in the Nutrition Facts) and see what one serving looks like.

There is something important to know about serving sizes. One portion of meat is equal to a deck of cards. If you typically put the equivalent of two or three or more decks of cards on your plate, does this mean that you can only have one deck of cards' worth of meat from now on at dinner? Not necessarily. It really depends on how many calories your body needs to maintain its weight, which varies from person to person. Most people tend to overdo it on the amount of protein they eat, and should stick to just one deck of cards' worth of meat or one serving of most foods.

Young suggests using a smaller plate to make the proper portion sizes look bigger at mealtime. Also, try loading up your plate with lower-calorie options, like leafy greens and other veggies to create the illusion of a full plate without overloading on calories. Since most veggies weigh in at only 25 calories per serving or less, it is a bit more difficult to get into trouble quickly with them as opposed to a serving of meat (3–4 ounces), which can pile on 150 to 200 calories in a hurry. 🆂🆁

| SKINNY RULE **52** | Don't Forget the Magic Meal |

Yes, there is one meal that is an absolute must for Skinny girls: breakfast.

Breakfast is the most important meal of the day, because it literally jump-starts your metabolism and gets your body going. Perhaps even more important, it provides the fuel (always remember, food is fuel) for your morning. As an added bonus, it will also help you perform and concentrate better at work or in school. In the National Weight Control Registry, the group that had lost and kept off 30 pounds for a year or more notes that breakfast is part of their everyday routine.

The everyday component is key. As with all the rules in this book, consistency is a crucial element because if you are just eating breakfast one day a week, you aren't putting this Skinny rule to work.

If you're not having breakfast every day or maybe not at all, start tomorrow and make it a daily goal. If you're not hungry when you wake up, you still need to eat breakfast. I know this sounds crazy—eat when you're not hungry? The reason you will need to do this is to get your body to adjust to eating breakfast. Over time, you will develop a morning appetite and you will actually wind up eating less food later in the day! The great part is that breakfast can be at whatever time works for you, not necessarily right when you first roll out of bed. If you're not hungry until, let's say, 10:00 a.m., make that your breakfast time. Maybe it's hard for you to make breakfast before you head out the door in the morning—that's okay, too. You can eat wherever you are in the midmorning.

While you can eat breakfast anywhere, you can't just eat anything. There is a perfect combination to strive for and that is a combination of carbohydrates and protein. This blend of nutrients will provide a belly-filling and longer-lasting energy boost than just having some carbohydrates alone. Here are some eat-anywhere breakfast solutions that deliver the ideal blend of nutrients and provide your body with ample energy to get your day off on the right foot.

You can eat breakfast like Jada Pinkett Smith. Jada shared with *Shape* magazine that she starts her day with a bowl of steel-cut oatmeal, topped with chicken and sesame seeds. Another great idea to try: 1 cup of plain yogurt topped with a cup of blueberries. If you're on the go and need something to eat in transit in the morning, opt for a protein bar, like Clif Bar, and a banana. If you have a little more time, scramble up 2 egg whites and 1 whole egg with diced onion and red pepper and serve with a slice of toasted whole-wheat bread. Or try making a fruit smoothie. Here is a favorite smoothie recipe of mine:

Skinny Smoothie

Serves 1

Ingredients

1 cup frozen fruit (e.g., blueberries, mango, banana, peaches)

1 cup plain yogurt

Splash of skim milk

1 scoop pure whey vanilla protein powder

Directions

1. Blend all the ingredients together until smooth.
2. Serve immediately.

Nutrition Facts (per serving)

360 calories, 1.5 grams fat, 0.5 grams saturated fat, 0 grams trans fat, 15 mg cholesterol, 290 mg sodium, 68 grams carbohydrates, 3 grams fiber, 50 grams sugar, 20 grams protein

Want to eat like the experts? Dr. David Katz, a leading researcher from Yale University told me his favorite breakfast is mixed berries (blueberries, blackberries, raspberries and strawberries) with a mix of whole-grain cereals (like Nature's Path Synergy) and some nonfat organic milk. As he says, "Manna from heaven!" A New York City–based registered dietitian and the registered dietitian behind the *Flat Belly Diet!* eating plan, Cynthia Sass, MPH, MA, RD, CSSD, likes to have one slice of whole-grain toast with almond butter, fresh in-season fruit and a soy latte. Then after the latte she switches to green, white, oolong, black or red tea. As for me, I love a bowl of whole-grain cereal (like Kamut or Cheerios), a banana or other fruit and a cup of black coffee. This is a frequent breakfast at our house—it's a hit with our younger little man and with my husband and me. (Of course, the coffee is just for the adults!)

Believe it or not, simply eating breakfast is even more important than what you eat, so don't delay; get started making breakfast part of your everyday eating routine! 🆂🆁

| SKINNY RULE 53 | Eat More Plant Foods |

The seemingly age-old advice is now coming from all around: Eat more fruits and vegetables. You will hear this very same Skinny rule from the government, nutrition professionals like myself and organizations like Produce for Better Health. Yet, as Dr. David Katz stated recently in the *Medscape Journal of Medicine,* "We eat fewer fruits and vegetables than we should. The reason there is a 'should' at all is the only reason that justifies any dietary guidance: food matters to health. That we are what we eat is as irrefutably true as it is inscrutably hard to see."

In the article, Dr. Katz further delved into just how poor fruit and vegetable intake is among Americans, referring to a study Kimmons and colleagues did with the Centers for Disease Control that compared fruit and vegetable intake to that of the advice in the USDA Food Guide Pyramid (otherwise known as MyPyramid). The findings were quite depressing across all demographics: Less than 1 percent of adolescents, roughly 2 percent of men and only

3½ percent of women met the guidelines for both fruits and vegetables. Even more depressing is that the low numbers were despite counting jam, jelly and orange juice as fruit, and both French fries and the ketchup poured over them, as vegetables. In fact, orange juice was the dominant fruit choice, and potatoes the dominant vegetable across all demographics.

A Skinny solution to increasing your fruit and vegetable intake is to have at least one fruit or vegetable at every meal and snack. *At breakfast:* Have a cup of plain yogurt topped with whole-grain cereal and a handful of blueberries. *For a snack:* Grab a banana or a handful of snow peas. *At lunch:* Have a baby spinach salad topped with veggies, some lean meat and chickpeas. *At dinner:* Make meat more of a side dish and let vegetables and fruit take center stage, filling up most of your plate, as compared to meat or starchy foods like rice.

This will mean upping the amount of fruits and vegetables that you purchase each week. Remember to select a variety of colors of fruits and vegetables to maximize the potential health benefits that comes from eating a range of fruits and vegetables.

When talking about fruits and vegetables, it is impossible not to bring up trying to buy locally. Food, especially produce, has quite the commute in many cases. On average, in the United States, produce travels 1,500 miles or more to get from farm to table. Of course, this affects the freshness factor, but transporting this food all around the globe via trucking, shipping and flying takes a toll on the environment as well. One example from the Natural Resources Defense Council: Every year, about 270 million pounds of grapes arrive in California, almost all of them shipped from Chile to Los Angeles—a 5,900-mile journey in cargo ships, which causes 7,000 tons of global-warming pollution each year!

Help the environment, know where your food is coming from and support your local economy by buying local. At one of my favorite websites, the Natural Resources Defense Council (www.nrdc.org), you can choose your state, the season and see what is fresh!

The NRDC identifies some of the "frequent fliers" as asparagus (Peru), bell peppers (the Netherlands), tomatoes (the Netherlands), blackberries (Chile), blueberries (Argentina), cherries (Chile), raspberries (Chile), peaches (Chile), nectarines (Chile) and papayas (Brazil).

As you boost your fruit and vegetable intake, take an environmentally friendly approach by trying to eat locally grown fresh fruits and vegetables most often. 🟢

SKINNY RULE 54	Take Control of Emotional Eating

For better or for worse, our moods definitely affect what we do and don't eat. We all seem to be a little different when it comes to how mood impacts our eating habits. Stress sends some people to the refrigerator; for others, it kills their appetite. Nonetheless, knowing how your moods impact your eating is an important first step to conquering this Skinny saboteur.

To figure out how your mood affects your eating, keep a diary of your food intake and feelings. Most important, be 100 percent honest. For example, if you grab a scoop of seconds at dinner, write it down or if you eat five handfuls of potato chips, write it down. Don't feel guilty! Awareness is what counts here. In addition to writing down what you ate, write down a few quick notes on your mood at the time— stressed out from a busy day at work, tired from a long day at the office, exhausted from chasing around your children, sad from a squabble with your boyfriend or husband. By being completely honest with yourself, you will be able to start to identify how emotions trigger eating patterns.

Once you know, you can create a plan to deal with it and curb your behaviors so your emotions don't control your appetite. Try these tried-and-true Skinny ways to curb emotional eating:

SAD? Instead of turning to a bag of potato chips or a carton of ice cream, put on your sneakers and go for a walk! If it's too cold to walk (no excuses), go to the mall!

TIRED? Grab a cup of warm green tea. The caffeine and flavonoids help to boost cognitive function and will give you a little extra energy, too.

UPSET? Try calling a friend or family member to talk about what is upsetting you. Oftentimes, just talking about what is on your mind will help ease the upset and make you feel better! After all, eating a bunch of brownies to cope with feeling glum will just leave you with a bellyache.

FRUSTRATED? Take a five-minute (or longer) yoga break to help balance your mind, body and spirit. If you have no clue how to do yoga, look for a yoga DVD to guide you along, like Mark Blanchard's Progressive Power Yoga.

HAPPY? Pamper yourself instead of using food to reward yourself. Give your nails a fresh coat of polish or really splurge and go for a massage!

BORED? If you fall victim to the nighttime munchies, do the Skinny thing and just go to bed. It's tough to eat while you're asleep!

Keep journaling your food intake and feelings in the process of trying some of the above tips and techniques to separate your emotions from food. It will help you to identify which ones work best for you. **SP**

Four

Skinny Cooking

<table>
<tr><td>

SKINNY
RULE
55

</td><td>

Keep Your Mouth Busy

</td></tr>
</table>

More and more, Americans are relying on restaurants as their dinner solution. Fast food expenditures shot up from 33 percent in 1970 to 45 percent in 2003. Meanwhile, obesity rates continue to climb. While restaurants are not totally to blame for our expanding waistlines, the frequency of eating out is still a huge factor in the overall balance of weight. And research shows that people who eat breakfast or dinner away from home are more likely to be overweight.

That said, cooking at home is something that Skinny people do often, and it is definitely a factor in keeping weight in check. A big perk you get from preparing meals at home is that you actually burn calories when cooking, to the tune of 85 calories per hour. You also burn another 35 calories in 15 minutes of washing dishes from your food preparation. If you were eating out an average of three times a week and started cooking at home two of those nights, you would burn approximately 120 calories twice a week for a total calorie burn of 240 calories per week and a yearly total of 12,480 calories, or about 3½ pounds' worth of calories! Remind yourself of these numbers the next time you think about grabbing the take-out menu and just picking up the phone to order a meal.

There is one more Skinny secret you must know when it comes to cooking at home. Have you ever grabbed a handful of chocolate chips while making cookies for the bake sale? Noshed on some bacon while cooking breakfast for a group? It is easy to do, which is where this Skinny rule comes in: Keep your mouth preoccupied while preparing foods. This means with something other than the food you are working with. A perfect solution is to chew on gum or drink a cup of tea. The simple act of keeping your taste buds preoccupied will help keep you from snacking while you are cooking and thereby unconsciously adding unwanted calories.

In just a half-ounce (less than a small handful), calories stack up quickly. Check it out:

- Chocolate chips add 70 calories and 4 grams of fat.
- Cheddar cheese (2 dice-size cubes) adds 57 calories and 4-plus grams of fat.
- Croutons add 66 calories and 2 or more grams of fat.

If you don't enjoy cooking or if you are cooking for just one or two, try for simple meal ideas, like grilled chicken seasoned with garlic powder, grilled sweet potatoes and sautéed green beans or a large bowl of dark leafy greens topped with veggies and diced turkey and cheese. There is no need to spend hours in the kitchen preparing food—just keep it simple, delicious and fresh! The less time it takes to prepare, the less time you have to keep your mouth busy before you eat. 🆂🆁

SKINNY RULE 56

Plan Your Plate

A simple Skinny secret is to customize your plate by filling it up with the right types of food. The key is to double the amount of vegetables you eat—aim to fill half your plate with them. Instead of cooking potatoes or rice with your meal, substitute an additional vegetable side dish. Steamed broccoli, a chopped salad or sautéed spinach are all good, easy choices that will fill you up and will save you hundreds of unwanted calories. Then, on the remaining half of the plate, fill one-quarter with fruit and one-quarter with protein. This Skinny way of filling your plate is a sure way to enjoy your meal while feeling satisfied.

Finally, fill your plate before you head to the table. Placing serving dishes on the table is too tempting and can easily lead to taking seconds and piling on extra, unnecessary calories.

Planning your plate naturally controls portion sizes, which is key to keeping your weight in check. I have been talking a lot about the calorie equation and the need to balance calories in and calories out; controlling portions is an important way to keeping caloric intake down. Even if you are filling your plate with all the right foods, if you are filling a platter-size dish instead of a dinner plate, you're overdoing it on portion sizes!

Skinny people are able to visualize healthy portion sizes. Here are some simple visual guides to follow for portion sizes:

- ½ cup pasta, rice, cereal, cooked vegetables or chopped fruit = ½ baseball.
- 3–4 ounces cooked meat = 1 deck of playing cards.
- 1 ounce snack foods like pretzels = a small handful.
- 1 ounce cheese cubes = 4 dice-size cubes.
- 2 tablespoons dressing = a shot glass.
- 1 medium fruit = a tennis ball.

For more information on portion sizes, go to www.mypyramid.gov.

One final Skinny tip: Downsize your plate to even further keep your portion size in check. The surface area of a dinner plate has ballooned by 36 percent since 1960. It's no wonder our waistlines have, too! 🆂🆁

SKINNY RULE 57

Spice It Up

Did you know that taste is one of the number one factors that determines what a person eats (price is the other main factor)? Sometimes people think that eating healthful foods doesn't taste good, yet Skinny girls know the secret to keeping their favorite foods full of flavor without adding tons of fat: using spices. In general, spices are an underutilized powerhouse in cooking because they provide few to no calories and pack in tons of flavor.

Stock your spice rack with the following spices and use these Skinny cooking secrets to jazz up your next meal:

GARLIC POWDER: Perhaps one of the most versatile spices. Season fresh tomatoes, vegetables, whole-wheat bread, chicken, steak, shrimp, soups…the list could go on and on.

ROSEMARY: One of my favorite spices, which actually belongs to the mint family. It adds great flavor to pizza, roasted vegetables, meat, poultry and stuffing.

PAPRIKA: A form of red pepper, some varieties are hotter than others, so be aware of the "hotness" of the one that you keep on hand. It is a perfect solution for adding mild flavor to egg dishes, sauces and salad dressings.

CHILI POWDER: This spice is actually a blend of spices, typically including chili peppers, garlic, paprika and oregano. The variety of flavors in chili powder makes it a wonderful addition to soups, meat and, of course, chili.

BASIL AND OREGANO: These classic Italian spices taste great in soups, sauces, on vegetables, in stews and on pizza. Try this quick recipe: Toss a chicken breast with extra virgin olive oil, basil and oregano. Transfer to a baking dish and bake at 350 degrees Fahrenheit for 20 to 30 minutes or until cooked thoroughly. This chicken tastes perfect on its own or when sliced on a salad or in a wrap.

CREOLE SEASONING: This adds a kick of flavor, so go easy the first time you try it. Use it to season a salmon filet and blacken it on a hot skillet. Serve with mango salsa.

GINGER: Sprinkle on chicken or steak and serve over steamed brown rice.

You can be adventurous and make your own spice blends! Taco and fajita seasoning is a breeze to make and tastes great on vegetables, too. Check out my husband's signature taco and fajita seasoning below (it also tastes great on corn!):

Skinny Taco and Fajita Seasoning

Ingredients

½ cup paprika

2 tablespoons coarse sea salt

2 tablespoons pure chili powder

1 tablespoon cracked black pepper

2 tablespoons garlic powder

1 tablespoon sugar

1 tablespoon onion powder

1 tablespoon dried cilantro

1½ teaspoons ground cumin

¾ teaspoon allspice

Directions

Combine the ingredients together and store in an airtight container.

Suggested uses: Season lean ground beef or chicken for fajitas, or sprinkle lightly on corn for a kicked-up cob. Adjust the amount you use to your taste preference.

Nutrition Facts (serving size: 1 teaspoon)

15 calories, 0 grams fat, 0 grams saturated fat, 0 grams trans fat, 0 mg cholesterol, 540 mg sodium, 3 grams carbohydrates, 1 gram fiber, less than 1 gram sugar, less than 1 gram protein ⓢⓡ

SKINNY RULE **58**

Try These Simple Skinny Substitutions

There are definite Skinny substitutions you can use in the kitchen to lighten up recipes and save calories while still enjoying your favorite foods. One of the simplest Skinny cooking tips to reduce the fat and calories in a recipe is just to cut the amount of total fat by a third. So if a recipe calls for three tablespoons of butter, take it right down to two tablespoons. Trust me, the recipe will still turn out A-Okay. Actually, you won't even notice that the extra fat is gone.

There are many other ways you can make the original recipe Skinny-friendly while preserving taste. Check out these Skinny secrets:

ALWAYS SUBSTITUTE a light version of products when available. For example, switch regular sour cream to light sour cream. For an even lighter option, use low-fat or fat-free, plain yogurt instead.

WHEN MAKING MAYONNAISE-BASED SALADS, sauces or dressing, substitute the light version for plain yogurt. The yogurt makes a fine stand-in because of its texture and tangy taste.

WHEN A RECIPE CALLS FOR VEGGIES, always add more! This works great with soups, stews and many side dishes.

FOR EVERY WHOLE EGG in a baking recipe use two egg whites, saving about 5 grams of total fat for each egg you replace.

INSTEAD OF CREAM, choose fat-free half 'n' half.

WHENEVER YOU'RE USING ITALIAN CHEESES, choose part-skim varieties like mozzarella and ricotta, instead of the whole-milk types.

Skinny Tip

Paulette Mitchell, the author of 14 cookbooks, including *The Complete 15-Minute Gourmet: Creative Cuisine Fast and Fresh,* shares a quick dressing recipe that uses nonfat yogurt instead of sour cream: Stir together a small carton of nonfat, plain yogurt, about ¼ cup fresh lime juice, sugar to taste and a dash of salt. Arrange a layer of greens on chilled plates. Top with chilled poached salmon steaks and lightly salted steamed and cooled green beans. Drizzle with the yogurt-lime dressing. Garnish with strips of lime zest.

SUBSTITUTE SOME OF THE HIGH-FAT INGREDIENTS when baking—for example, use applesauce, apple butter or yogurt in place of oil in a muffin or cookie recipe (suggested by Dana Angelo White and Toby Amidor, registered dietitians and nutrition experts for www.healthyeats.com).

REPLACE HALF THE CHEESE in a homemade mac 'n' cheese or quesadilla recipe with low-fat cottage cheese. (Quick tip: Blend the cottage cheese first until it is creamy and smooth.)

SUBSTITUTE CHICKEN BROTH FOR OIL in some recipes. This handy tip, from a cousin of mine, Kristine Schoembs, helps her maintain a healthy weight. Her homemade pesto recipe has very little oil in it: 2 cups fresh basil leaves, ½ cup chicken broth, ¼ cup grated Parmesan cheese, 1 tablespoon extra virgin olive oil and 2–3 garlic cloves. Put all these ingredients in a food processor and blend. You won't even miss all the oil! Pour it over meat, chicken, fish or veggies or add it to pasta.

Now, I have to say, while making recipe substitutions is a great way to enjoy foods in a lighter way, eating healthy and living a Skinny life is still all about balance. Let me share with you a perfect example. Recently my sister-in-law, Gretchen, made a delicious Asiago chicken pasta dish and I immediately asked her for the recipe. In the same breath my husband chimed in, "Don't you dare try to lighten this up. When you make it, please follow the recipe as is!" There may be certain family favorites or indulgent dishes that just need to be left alone and enjoyed as is. Try reserving these recipes as more of an occasional "treat." These substitutions will help you make healthier meals the rest of the time. 🆂🆁

SKINNY RULE 59	Don't Follow the Recipe

Although it is tempting to stick to a recipe exactly, the truth of the matter is there is a lot of wiggle room in most recipes. I think Rachael Ray demonstrates this best with her time-saving tips on how to measure when cooking. For instance, for a teaspoon of garlic powder, Rachael advises just to sprinkle a little bit in the palm of your hand and then add it to your dish. There isn't a need (at least for most recipes) to be too concerned about measuring precisely. That's also true when it comes to the ingredient list. There are many ways you can take traditional recipes and lighten them up while still making them taste equally delicious!

Chef Eric Khron, who recommends creating your own recipes from scratch, states, "Healthy eating is not about replicating a specific recipe, but creating a new dish." To do this, Khron suggests that you start by choosing your vegetable, protein and starch. Ideally, these will be seasonal items found in your local grocery store or market. Then choose a cooking method for each item: sautéed broccoli, braised chicken breasts and steamed couscous, for example.

Once you've got the basics down and are comfortable creating your own meals, Chef Khron recommends that you "start to have fun with your meal. Choose a nationality, a favorite holiday or any other theme." Then use your theme to season your dish appropriately; for instance, Indian spices, wintery nutmeg and cinnamon or citrus zest.

Getting away from a recipe and putting together your own original meal is both rewarding and healthy.

Here is a tasty recipe from Chef Khron. Enjoy!

Skinny Zucchini Omelet

Serves 4
A fun summer and fall dish.

Ingredients

2 pounds zucchini, shredded

1 teaspoon baking powder

1 cup whole-wheat flour

8 beaten egg whites

2 ounces feta cheese

Directions

1. In a mixing bowl, combine zucchini, baking powder, flour and beaten eggs. Mix.

2. Pour this mixture onto a hot, flat-top pan, like a cast-iron skillet. Then transfer to a preheated oven at 350 degrees Fahrenheit and bake for 15 minutes.

3. Turn the broiler on, brown the top and remove from the oven. Cut into fourths and flip.

4. Finish by sprinkling with feta cheese.

Nutrition Facts (per serving)

210 calories, 4 grams fat, 2.5 grams saturated fat, 0 grams trans fat, 15 mg cholesterol, 410 mg sodium, 31 grams carbohydrates, 6 grams fiber, 5 grams sugar, 16 grams protein 🆂🆁

SKINNY RULE
60

Cook Like a Celebrity...Chef

Robin Miller, host of the Food Network's *Quick Fix Meals* and author of *Robin Rescues Dinner*, weighs in with her top five Skinny cooking tips and techniques:

1. **LIGHTEN UP** homemade salad dressing and pesto by using low sodium, fat-free chicken or vegetable broth instead of most of the oil called for in the recipe (keep about 2–3 teaspoons of the total amount of oil and substitute broth for the rest).

2. **SWAP WHITE BEANS** for chickpeas in hummus and white beans or canned asparagus for half the avocado in guacamole before puréeing until smooth.

3. **MAKE PARFAITS** with layers of nonfat yogurt, fresh fruit and granola or crumbled vanilla or chocolate wafer cookies. Or sweeten part-skim ricotta cheese with vanilla extract and use that instead of yogurt in the same parfaits.

4. **COAT BONELESS, SKINLESS CHICKEN BREASTS** with honey mustard and then coat with a mixture of instant oats and salt-free garlic and herb seasoning. Spray pan with cooking spray. Bake at 375 degrees Fahrenheit for 25–30 minutes, until golden brown and cooked through (no deep frying!).

5. **STUFF FLOUR TORTILLAS** with a mixture of fat-free refried beans, cooked brown rice and prepared salsa. Roll up and place side-by-side in a baking dish. Bake at 375 degrees Fahrenheit for 15 minutes, until tortillas are golden and filling is hot. Top with nonfat sour cream, salsa and cilantro before serving. 🄢

SKINNY RULE 61
Think of the Freezer as Your Friend

Hopefully, all this talk about cooking is getting you excited about rolling up your sleeves, putting on an apron and heading to the kitchen! As you cook more at home, you will wind up with more leftovers. Some people love leftovers; others do not. Even if you don't mind leftovers, eating the same thing for too many days in a row gets a bit boring. A Skinny solution for leftovers is to freeze at least some of your leftovers for a later date! This will keep your taste buds from getting bored with what you made and ensures that you'll always have a healthy meal at the ready for when you need it.

Here are a few quick tips to follow when you fill up your freezer with leftovers, so it doesn't become a maddening mess. The first step is to label whatever you put in the freezer. If you are using plastic or glass storage containers, write the contents on a piece of masking tape and then tape the label to the container. If you are using freezer bags, be sure to mark the bag with a permanent marker. Since foods do not last in the freezer forever, it is important to date the foods so you know when the food was made. Although food will last in a freezer for a long time, for maximum quality, a good rule of thumb is to try to use up what is in your freezer within three to four months.

Another Skinny solution when you start stocking up your freezer is to keep a freezer list. You may be wondering, What the heck is a freezer list? Basically, it is a list of what you actually have in the freezer. When you put something in the freezer, add it to the list with the date and, just as important, when you take something out of the freezer, remove it from the list. This will help you keep track of what you have in the freezer and will be a real time-saver.

Other freezer-friendly tips: Designate areas of your freezer for particular items. Try using the freezer door for frozen vegetables and fruit (Skinny foods that should be on hand at all times). Here is a tip I learned from my mom: Take clear plastic bins and use one for chicken, one for beef, one for leftover side dishes and so on. These bins become the place where you store the corresponding food items. It's a great way to easily keep everything in your freezer organized, so you can dig out whatever you need in a hurry. Notice that there isn't much space left for ice cream! ⓢⓡ

SKINNY RULE
62

Reinvent Your Leftovers

Next time you're not sure what to do with last night's chicken, try this Skinny strategy for leftovers: Reinvent them! Rather than thinking, Oh, no—another night of grilled chicken, turn the grilled chicken into a quesadilla filled with fresh salsa, corn, avocado and shredded cheese with light sour cream to dip it in. Check out these exciting ways to reinvent what you couldn't finish at a meal so it doesn't wind up getting pushed to the back of your refrigerator and growing mold.

GRILLED CHICKEN: Cube the chicken into bite-size pieces. Then make wraps for lunch using whole-wheat tortillas and filling the wrap with fresh vegetables, like tomato slices and baby spinach.

PASTA: Slice a zucchini, summer squash and any other vegetables that need to be used up. Place them in a sauté pan, add a small amount of extra virgin olive oil and season with basil, garlic and oregano. Sauté the vegetables until they are tender. Next drain and rinse a can of dark red kidney beans and toss them in and warm. Lastly, add your left over pasta and heat until warm. Serve with a small amount of grated Parmesan cheese. YUM! (Note: Adjust the amount of vegetables that you add, depending on how much pasta you have left over.)

STEAK: Slice a sweet onion and sauté the onion with a small amount of extra virgin olive oil until tender. Slice the steak into thin strips and heat thoroughly with the onion. Place on a whole-wheat roll and sprinkle on top a small amount of shredded cheddar cheese.

DELI MEAT: You can do so many different things with deli meat! Try slicing deli turkey or ham and adding it to your next pasta salad.

RICE: Have brown rice with dinner on Monday night and transform it into yummy stir-fried rice for Tuesday night! Check out my yummy stir-fried rice recipe in Skinny Rule #63, Keep a Recipe Notebook. This recipe is a great way to use up extra veggies, too!

VEGGIES: Try this Skinny soup recipe of my grandma's: Take chicken stock and dice up leftover veggies of any type. Even stir in leftover rice and chicken for a heartier soup. Season the soup to taste with garlic powder and black pepper. YUM!

MASHED POTATOES: If you overdid it on the amount of mashed potatoes that you made, transform them the next night with some veggies and lean ground beef! Cook the lean ground beef in a pan until done. Transfer to a pie plate then top with veggies, like green beans and diced carrots, and finish with your leftover mashed potatoes. Bake at 350 degrees Fahrenheit until everything is heated thoroughly. Enjoy! SR

SKINNY
RULE
63

Keep a Recipe Notebook

This is a Skinny way to keep a log of your favorite recipes, meals, menus and even bottles of wine. You can purchase something fancy that has dividers, storage folders and matching recipe cards *or* you can keep it simple and just use a notebook. The reason this works is because you are building your own tried-and-true book of favorite recipes. And remember: Simply cooking at home as opposed to eating out is a smart Skinny choice—you burn calories while cooking and you will likely eat fewer calories than you would have eaten out. As a side note, this makes a great wedding gift, too!

Here are some of my favorite Skinny recipes. Use them to start your own recipe notebook:

Skinny Fried Rice

Serves 4

Ingredients

2 teaspoons vegetable oil

2½ cups assorted cooked vegetables

4 egg whites

2 tablespoons soy sauce, lite

1 teaspoon sesame oil

1 cup cooked brown rice

2 tablespoons chopped onion

Directions

1. In a large skillet or wok, heat oil and add veggies and chopped onion. Cook until the onions are tender.

2. Move the veggies to the sides of the pan, add the egg whites in the middle and scramble the eggs.

3. Once the egg whites begin to solidify, add the soy sauce, sesame oil and rice. Toss to combine ingredients and warm rice through.

Nutrition Facts (per serving)

130 calories, 4 grams fat, 0.5 grams saturated fat, 0 grams trans fat, 0 mg cholesterol, 320 mg sodium, 17 grams carbohydrates, 2 grams fiber, 1 gram sugar, 7 grams protein

Skinny Crab and Corn Chowder

Yield: 12 one-cup servings

Ingredients

1 teaspoon olive oil

1 tablespoon butter

3 red potatoes, chopped

2 stalks celery, chopped

2 small red peppers, chopped

1 bay leaf

2 tablespoons all-purpose flour

2 cups low-sodium chicken stock

1 quart fat-free milk

3 cups frozen corn kernels

8 ounces crabmeat

Salt

Pepper

Directions

1. Heat oil and butter and add potatoes, celery and peppers. Add bay leaf.

2. Sauté veggies for about five minutes and then sprinkle in the flour.

3. Cook for a few minutes, stirring continuously and then add in the broth and stir to combine.

4. Add in the milk, stir to combine and then bring to a boil. Once the mixture boils, let it bubble about one minute more. (Stir occasionally through this process.)

5. Add in the corn and crabmeat and simmer for five minutes. Add salt and pepper as needed.

Tip for a thicker soup: Let the soup continue to simmer until it has reduced by about a quarter.

Nutrition Facts (per serving)

170 calories, 2.5 grams fat, 1 gram saturated fat, 0 grams trans fat, 15 mg cholesterol, 290 mg sodium, 29 grams carbohydrates, 3 grams fiber, 7 grams sugar, 10 grams protein 🆂🆁

SKINNY RULE **64**

Stock Your Kitchen with These Must-Have Skinny Tools

You don't need a state-of-the-art kitchen to cook healthy foods, but having a few simple tools on hand will make food prep a breeze and aid in creating healthy dishes.

Here are a few essential gadgets that must make their way into your kitchen (if they're not there already).

THE FIRST MUST-HAVE is a garlic press. Peeling garlic is just a sticky mess and a garlic press eliminates that.

EVERY SKINNY KITCHEN needs a mini food processor. This is the perfect solution for chopping up food, blending hummus or puréeing soups. The mini version is easier to handle than its bulky and large counterpart.

TWO MUST-HAVE COOKING TOOLS are a rice cooker and a wok. The rice cooker prepares tasty rice more simply than conventional methods, plus it keeps it warm until dinner is ready. A wok creates such a quick meal solution that, although bulky, every kitchen should have one. It is perfect for stir-frying, cooking vegetables and sautéing rice noodles, too.

AN OLIVE OIL SPRAYER is another great tool! (I actually think a salad dressing bottle that has a sprayer or a marinade bottle makes a better olive oil sprayer than the types that are marketed to do so.) A sprayer is so helpful to have on hand because when you pour olive oil onto a pan you likely add more than you actually need to cook. While olive oil is a heart-healthy food, it still comes with a hefty calorie price tag of about 120 calories per tablespoon (which equals three teaspoons) and 14 grams of fat. The sprayer we use in our kitchen sprays about a quarter of a teaspoon with each spray or about 10 calories and just under one gram of fat per spray. When you get your sprayer home, check how much comes out with each spray so you can easily know how much you are adding during cooking.

A BLENDER for making smoothies. Store-bought smoothies tend to be loaded with syrups and sugars and may not even have much fruit in them at all. Having a blender will allow you to whip up your own delicious (and Skinnier) smoothies regularly. You can even add an immersion blender to your collection—it is perfect for smoothies and puréeing sauces and soups.

MAKING PIZZA AT HOME is easy and in most cases healthier than purchased pizza and all you will need are a pizza stone and some toppings and dough. The great part about making pizza at home is that you can use whole-wheat dough, control the type and amount of cheese you use and choose your own toppings!

A CEDAR PLANK often comes with a recipe book, but some Skinny favorites to cook on it include roasted veggies and salmon. The cedar infuses a delicious flavor into your cooking and is a simple and tasty way to prepare foods a little out of the ordinary.

Equipping your kitchen with these Skinny gadgets and cooking tools will allow you to take another step to living a healthier, Skinnier life. 🅢

| SKINNY RULE **65** | Be a Star in Your Kitchen |

There are so many kitchen reality shows, but here's the good news: You don't need to be on a reality cooking TV show to be acclaimed as a great chef. You can be a star in your own kitchen! My guess is you have cookbooks stashed somewhere in your kitchen that may be collecting dust. If that is the case, getting out the cookbooks is a great place to start. Grab some of those cookbooks and slowly challenge yourself to try some new recipes. Being a great cook doesn't have to be complicated and, remember, you don't have to follow the recipe exactly. But dusting off the cookbooks will inspire you to try something new and make you feel a little bit more like a cooking star. This Skinny rule is especially important if you often find yourself saying, "I have no idea what to cook for dinner."

If you don't have a lot of cookbooks around, no worries! Head to the library and borrow some cookbooks or go to a bookstore and treat yourself to a new one. Even ask a friend if you can borrow a cookbook for a while. Another great place to look for recipes is the Internet. There are plenty of websites with delicious recipes to choose from. One of my favorites is www.foodnetwork.com. That site is loaded with great recipes from a variety of chefs. I especially love that www.foodnetwork.com provides a "healthy eating" option where you can click to get links to healthy recipes. Many of the recipes are actually created by the Food Network chefs who are registered dietitians (RDs) and nutrition experts. You can also search by particular food item to find recipes. This is particularly helpful if you are trying to figure out a way to get rid of something that is sitting in your cupboard or refrigerator waiting to be used up.

One of the other greatest recipe resources is family! Grandmothers and mothers can be walking recipe boxes. My grandmothers, mom and mother-in-law have shared many of their tasty recipes with me over the years. This is a great way to learn new cooking techniques as well.

For additional recipes, subscribe to a cooking magazine. A lot of health magazines have recipes in them every month, too. Some of my personal favorites include *Rachael Ray, Fitness, Shape, Women's Health, Eating Well,* and *Cooking Light.* Next time someone asks you what you want for a birthday or a holiday, ask for the gift of a subscription to a magazine of your choice and you will have new meal ideas delivered to your door on a monthly basis! That will surely help keep your taste buds interested and make you a star in your kitchen.

Then, when you discover a new recipe that you love, add it to your recipe notebook. This way you will have the recipe right on hand to whip up the next time around. Also, be sure you note any adjustments or substitutions that you made because, remember, there is no need to follow the recipe to the letter. Be creative! 🔘

SKINNY RULE 66

Be Your Own Sous-Chef

In our kitchen, the sous-chef is the one who does all the prep work. Oftentimes, I am the sous-chef and my husband is the head chef, as he is an amazing cook.

Even if you don't have someone to work under you (so to speak) in the kitchen, you can be your own sous-chef—and being your own sous-chef is a helpful Skinny rule, especially when you're new to cooking. What does it mean to be your own sous-chef? Essentially, you will do all the prep work to make your cooking adventure go smoothly. This starts right when you are getting ready to make a meal. Take a look at your recipe and get everything ready to go that you will need. Measure out the various ingredients, chop up what you need to, get your pans out, preheat the oven and so on. This will make preparing your meal go much more smoothly. It will also help you be the star in your kitchen—you will look and feel more like a cooking show host when you aren't running around your kitchen with no plan in place.

If you're really busy, start preparing food right when you get home from the grocery store. Instead of just tossing the produce in the crisper drawer, put it all on the countertop, wash what needs to be washed, chop what needs to be chopped and cook what needs to be cooked. We do this during farmers' market season. My husband and our little guys go to the farmers' market and get a bunch of fresh produce, then sous-chef mommy (me, that is) gets to work in the evening once the boys are in bed. I will snip and prepare the green beans, shuck the corn on the cob and rinse them so they are ready to go at dinnertime the next night. I will also wash and slice a bowl of peaches so we can enjoy them easily at breakfast the next morning. And my favorite—I'll scrub and boil beets, then cube them so we can add them to salads or have them as a side dish with our meal. While this process takes a little bit of time, it saves time in the long run and it's really worth it. It makes having healthy foods at every meal a reality. 🆂🆁

SKINNY RULE 67

Stock Your Pantry with Skinny Essentials

Have you ever gone to cook something and not had all the ingredients? There is nothing more frustrating! Keeping a well-stocked pantry will make Skinny cooking a breeze by simply keeping essential ingredients on hand to prepare tasty and healthy dishes. Notice that in this section I keep talking about tasty dishes. A Skinny secret is that healthy foods can taste just as good as their higher-fat counterparts, if not better. It is all about using the right ingredients.

FRESH GARLIC: One of the most flavorful and versatile vegetables there is. Think green, look for local sources of fresh garlic at farm stands and always keep a couple of cloves of garlic on hand to add to vegetables, chicken, fish, marinades, dipping sauces and more.

HEART-HEALTHY OILS: Keep a variety of oils in stock, including extra virgin olive oil, light olive oil, canola oil, sunflower oil and sesame oil. Having a variety of oils will enable you to enhance dishes with flavor as you see fit. When you're looking to add little to no flavor to a dish, opt for canola or light olive oil. For a nutty flavor, choose sunflower or sesame oil. And for a rich olive oil flavor, choose the purest of the oils—extra virgin olive oil, which comes from the first press of olives. Just remember that you should use these oils in moderation to reach your Skinny goals—using an oil sprayer will help (see Skinny Rule #64).

VINEGARS: White-wine, red-wine, balsamic and white balsamic vinegar are all Skinny cooking must-haves. They all add wonderful flavors to dishes with virtually no calories. White, red-wine and balsamic vinegars are perfect for salad dressings and marinades. You can use white and red-wine vinegars in a variety of sauces as well. Here is a favorite Skinny secret to add flavor to salads and veggies without adding calories. In a small saucepan, place 4 ounces of balsamic vinegar, let it reduce to half and then drizzle on salads or veggies. YUM!

WHOLE-WHEAT FLOUR: It provides more nutrients and fiber than its traditional counterpart. As an added bonus, the fiber helps to keep you full, compared to plain old white flour. In any recipe that calls for flour, try replacing at least half the flour with whole wheat and work your way up to cooking with 100 percent whole-wheat flour. Gradually working up to 100 percent whole-wheat baking will allow your taste buds to adjust on your way to using 100 percent whole wheat. Eventually, like me, you can just stop keeping white flour on hand. I even use 100 percent whole-wheat flour now to make cakes for special occasions—and they are still crowd pleasers.

HONEY: It has more sweetening power than white sugar and it can virtually replace white sugar in any recipe. A drizzle of honey is perfect in tea, on shrimp before grilling or even in baked goods. Use 8 ounces of honey for every 10 ounces of sugar the recipe calls for.

GROUND FLAXSEED: Full of heart-healthy and belly-slimming fat, flax is a great addition to many dishes and can be added to hot cereal like oatmeal. You can even add it to meatballs, burgers and rice dishes. It will simply add a little texture and a light nutty flavor, while upping the nutritional quality of your recipes.

SEASONED SALT: A perfect Skinny way to add flavor to your foods without adding fat or calories! That's because seasoned salt is mixed with other herbs and spices, so it offers less sodium per teaspoon as compared to regular table salt. Keep in mind that it still contains sodium so you don't have a green light to go crazy with it, especially if you are sensitive to sodium or have high blood pressure.

PANKO BREAD CRUMBS: This bread crumb variety, common in Japanese cuisine, is a terrific Skinny ingredient for making foods like chicken fingers that taste fried even when they are just pan-fried or baked! Panko bread crumbs are crunchy and delicious. Coat chicken tenders in them and then bake or pan-fry them with a little extra virgin olive oil until thoroughly cooked. Look for them in Asian markets and large grocery stores. ⓢ

SKINNY
RULE
68

Feature the Right Foods in Your Fridge

I checked in with some nutrition and health experts to see what foods they recommend featuring in your refrigerator. Consider what the director and co-founder of the Yale Prevention Research Center, Dr. David Katz, suggests: "There is no food that must be in the fridge at all times. Here are some I think should be featured frequently: salmon, spinach and/or broccoli, berries, nonfat milk or plain yogurt and organic mixed greens." Here's why:

FOR NONVEGETARIANS: Keep salmon on hand because it is a highly nutritious source of protein and omega-3s.

VEGGIES TO FEATURE: Spinach and/or broccoli because they are among the most nutritious of all foods when nutrients are measured relative to calories.

BERRIES: Berries are part of Dr. Katz's complete breakfast (see Skinny Rule #52), plus they are highly nutritious and delicious.

ORGANIC MIXED GREENS: Dr. Katz believes that salad should be part of every dinner. He suggests opting for the prewashed mixes to make it easy.

Cynthia Sass, MPH, MA, RD, CSSD, New York City–based registered dietitian and nutrition expert of the *Flat Belly Diet!* recommends stocking your fridge with pesto, water, dark chocolate and hummus. Here's how and why:

PESTO: Make sure it's a pesto made with nutritious and delicious extra virgin olive oil. Sass explains that pesto is "an awesome source of antioxidants and heart-healthy fat, and a little goes a long way." Her tip is to use pesto to spruce up steamed veggies, whole-grain pasta, quinoa or other whole grains.

WATER: Sass explains that water is the most important nutrient of all; it is what 60 percent of our bodies are made of. Sass recommends keeping a pitcher of filtered water in the fridge at all times. "Keeping it in the fridge in a pitcher helps the environment (no empty plastic bottles) and if it's the first thing you see when you open the fridge you'll be more likely to drink it," she explains.

DARK CHOCOLATE: This is loaded with good fats and antioxidants, which help slash the risk of heart disease, says Sass. Registered dietitian Elisa Zied, MS, RD, CDN, spokesperson for the American Dietetic Association and author of *Nutrition at Your Fingertips* and *Feed Your Family Right!* suggests that consuming a small amount of high-quality dark chocolate every day can keep you satisfied so you won't go overboard.

HUMMUS: This is a great way to incorporate more beans into your diet! Keeping hummus in the fridge will help you get the three cups of beans per week recommended by registered dietitians. For a switch from traditional hummus, which is made with chickpeas, try making (or buying) some made with black beans, edamame and other legumes. It's a perfect dip for raw veggies or a mayo alternative for sandwiches.

In addition to these great recommendations, dedicate some shelf space to these healthy essentials:

FLAXSEED AND/OR FISH OIL both provide health-promoting omega fats and are perfect to drizzle on salad, add to smoothies or even just take a quick spoonful to gain all the health benefits. Plus, as an added benefit, one tablespoon of the oil is equal to taking, in some cases, 12 or more of the pill form of omega-3 fats.

100 PERCENT FRUIT JUICE is another good item to have on hand. It is a great addition to a glass of water to add a little flavor and keep your taste buds interested. Great for smoothies, too.

KEEP NATURAL ALMOND AND/OR PEANUT BUTTER on hand, which is tasty to have with fruit like a pear or an apple, for a PB and J sandwich or to spread lightly on some whole-grain crackers for a snack. The natural butters don't have all the added preservatives and sugar of the traditional kind. Most need to be refrigerated.

Try keeping an ongoing shopping list on the refrigerator door so when you run out of one of these staple items you remember to pick it up on the next shopping trip. This way you will make sure that you always have your Skinny essentials at the ready! ⓢⓡ

| SKINNY RULE **69** | Try These Simple Skinny Meal Concepts |

ere is a Skinny rule that you must keep in mind: You have to have at least a handful of what I like to call "meal concepts" up your sleeve. Meal concepts are meals that come together effortlessly and are made from the staple items you keep around the house. They are meals that you can easily whip up on nights when you don't feel like cooking. These Skinny meal concepts will help you have quick, tasty and healthy meals ready in minutes!

These meal concepts can be scaled up or down, depending on how many people you are serving. Too many times I hear people complain, "I hate cooking for just the two of us, or just me." That's just a Skinny excuse—truth is, there's no need to make it complicated! I spent years cooking just for one and then just for two, so I know exactly how you feel. But, trust me, with simple meal concepts you'll have a meal ready to go with little effort and in no time at all!

No cookbook is necessary for these Skinny meal concepts:

ON THE GRILL: Grilled steak or pork seasoned with sea salt and cracked pepper with a side of grilled asparagus, served with a whole-wheat dinner roll.

READY IN MINUTES: In a sauté pan, add a small amount of extra virgin olive oil. Then add boneless, skinless chicken tenders and season with garlic (fresh or ground). Sauté until the chicken is thoroughly cooked. Add in a few handfuls of baby spinach, cook until the spinach is wilted and serve warm with a drizzle of balsamic vinegar.

SALMON BURGERS: In a food processor purée a 3-ounce salmon filet, then stir in a small handful of panko bread crumbs. Press into a patty and cook in a sauté pan until the salmon is cooked thoroughly. Serve the burger on a whole-wheat roll and, as a delicious addition, top with sliced avocado. On the side, serve it with a baked sweet potato and fresh spinach salad.

VEGGIE PASTA: Prepare whole-wheat pasta according to the package instructions and set pasta aside. In a sauté pan, add a small amount of extra virgin olive oil and sauté a handful of sliced summer squash and zucchini with a few cloves of garlic. Add in the pasta and top with shredded Parmesan cheese.

Skinny Tip

Triathlete Christa Winslow knows that protein and nutrients are essential for her athletic lifestyle, but she keeps her dinners simple and easy to make. As she explains, she always has a salad loaded with lots of fresh, raw, colorful veggies, including dark greens like spinach, romaine lettuce, tomatoes, peppers and onions. To save time, she makes enough salad for at least two meals and sometimes adds some dried cranberries and nuts for extra crunch. Along with the salad, she'll grill salmon, stuffed filet of flounder, steak or chicken. Her favorite side dish is brown rice and for flavor she sticks with herbs and always cooks with olive oil to get some "good fat" into the meal.

QUESADILLA: Fill a whole-wheat tortilla with a small amount of shredded cheese, chopped fresh veggies and whatever leftover meat you have on hand (e.g., steak or chicken). In a skillet, heat until the cheese is melted and the tortilla shell is lightly browned. Serve with a side of light sour cream and salsa. Enjoy a salad made from dark greens, like romaine lettuce, for a side dish.

ASIAN CHICKEN: Prepare rice noodles according to the package instructions. In a skillet, cook cubed chicken, seasoned with a small amount of sesame oil, ground ginger and garlic powder. Once the chicken is cooked, toss in a handful of frozen or fresh snap peas. Then add a handful of rice noodles and drizzle with low-sodium soy sauce.

No excuses! Put away the take-out menus and make a quick and delicious meal using these Skinny meal concepts. Don't think of these concepts as recipes, but as simple "formulas" for a meal, which can be easily adapted to work with whatever food you have on hand. Give them a try. 🆂🆁

SKINNY RULE 70 — Make Skinny Food Fun

How can foods like baby spinach, carrots, apples, oranges, whole-wheat breads, boneless, skinless chicken breasts and low-fat milk be fun? There are so many ways! Somehow Skinny food has gotten a stigma as boring. Yet there are seemingly endless ways that you can make even healthy food fun. This is something that Skinny girls know and use to get into those skinny jeans.

Making food fun can vary from experimenting with new recipes to being creative with old favorites; both are certain to add new flavor and keep food fun! If you need more suggestions on how to make food fun, see Skinny Rule #65, Be a Star in Your Kitchen. And if you need help on revamping recipes, go back to Skinny Rule #58, Try These Simple Skinny Substitutions.

Make It a Social Gathering

One way to make cooking fun is to cook with family members and friends. Just being in the kitchen working with someone makes the process of cooking much less like a chore and more like a social gathering. Plus, in the process, you can pick up cooking tips and new recipes. Recently, my mom and I had a few marathon cooking nights where we made homemade peach jelly, spaghetti sauce, canned tomatoes and frozen peaches. My mom had gone to a farmers' market to stock up on peaches, tomatoes and the veggies for the spaghetti sauce, and then we prepared everything together at her house. As a Skinny bonus, this makes having fresh foods and healthier foods on hand so simple, you can control how the foods are prepared and, perhaps best of all, you know where the food came from.

You don't need to plan a marathon session to put this tip into action. Invite a group of friends over for a girls' night of cooking and eating. You can catch up over some wine, while experimenting in the kitchen. Instead of going out to dinner with your boyfriend, cook together! Food often tastes best when it's shared, so don't be afraid to make cooking a social event.

Throw a Progressive Dinner

Another way to make food fun is to have a progressive dinner. Get a group of friends or family onboard and have every house plan a different course of your meal. Then you go from house to house, enjoying your meal. When you are planning your dinner, remember to keep the portions at each course small, as you'll be slowly eating your way through dinner as you progress from house to house. Another reason this is a Skinny rule is that, even though you will be eating throughout the evening, you will be eating slowly, giving your brain time to signal, *Hey! I'm full.*

Remember, it takes about 20 minutes for your belly to signal to your brain that you have had enough to eat.

Try this Skinny progressive dinner menu: *Soup:* Vegetable soup; *Salad:* Baby spinach with beets, feta and toasted walnuts; *Entrée:* Grilled marinated pork tenderloin; *Sides:* Baked sweet potatoes and sliced tomatoes with pesto; and *Dessert:* Coffee with berry yogurt parfaits.

Give Traditional Foods a Twist

Jazzing up traditional foods with a new twist is another great way to make food fun. Rather than just serving brown rice as a side dish, why not brown rice sautéed with mixed vegetables? Or instead of having a cup of yogurt for breakfast, try layering in a serving dish yogurt, diced fruit and whole-grain cereal—a fresh new way to enjoy yogurt! If you're bored with the usual salads, try adding fruit to your salad, like mandarin oranges, dried cranberries, sliced strawberries or grilled pears.

Another favorite way to make foods fun is by serving them on skewers—this works great for fruit, grilled fish and veggie kabobs. You can even make sandwiches on a stick. Here are two simple skewer recipes to help you make healthy foods fun! (A quick side note on skewers: For safety reasons [especially when serving to children], take kitchen scissors and snip the sharp end off the skewer before serving.)

Skinny Sandwich on a Stick

Serves 2

Ingredients

2 slices thick, crusty, whole-grain bread
4 ounces thickly sliced roasted turkey breast
cherry tomatoes
chunks of pickles
grapes
wooden skewers

Directions

On the wooden skewers, place alternating cubes of bread, turkey, tomatoes, pickles and grapes. (Plan for 2 ounces of turkey per serving and 1 slice of cubed bread per serving.)

Serving suggestion: Serve with honey mustard as a dipping sauce.

Nutrition Facts (per serving)

180 calories, 3 grams fat, 0 grams saturated fat, 0 grams trans fat, 25 mg cholesterol, 620 mg sodium, 25 grams carbohydrates, 3 grams fiber, 8 grams sugar, 15 grams protein

Skinny Chicken Kabobs

Serves 2

Ingredients

6 ounces chicken breast

chunks of pineapple

chunks of mango

chunks of roasted red peppers

wooden skewers

Directions

1. Soak the skewers in water for 10 to 15 minutes before using. This prevents the skewers from burning when on the grill.

2. Cut chicken breast, fruit and peppers into large cubes and alternate on skewers. (Plan for about 3 ounces of chicken per kabob and load up the rest with fruit and vegetables.)

3. Grill until fruit and veggies are tender and chicken is cooked thoroughly.

Serving suggestion: Serve over whole-grain couscous or steamed brown rice.

Nutrition Facts (per serving)

290 calories, 3 grams fat, 1 gram saturated fat, 0 grams trans fat, 99 mg cholesterol, 114 mg sodium, 27 grams carbohydrates, 3 grams fiber, 21 grams sugar, 41 grams protein ⑤®

Five

Skinny Parties and Travel

SKINNY RULE 71	Go to a Party Full

This may sound loony, but it's true: Skinny girls go to a party full or, at the very least, have a satisfying snack beforehand so they aren't ravenous. Why does this work? At a party, you never know what kind of food is going to be offered and how it was prepared. Plus, let's be honest: Parties tend to be a recipe for un-Skinny disaster. Usually there is drinking involved as well as foods with a heavy calorie price tag that you likely don't eat on a regular basis. If you enter into that situation famished, you are most likely going to overeat.

So before you leave for your next get-together, have a small meal or a snack to take the edge off your hunger; think of it as a "mini meal." This will set you up to face the party environment in a more controlled manner. Sure, you will still enjoy some of your favorite party foods, but you will be able to do so without overindulging in fattening foods, and as a bonus, it will allow you to spend more time socializing. Don't forget: A very important Skinny rule is splurging (see Skinny Rule #16), so don't mistake this rule for eating only veggies and drinking water at a party! What fun would that be?

For your preparty snack, try these ideas:

- an apple and a part-skim mozzarella cheese stick
- whole-grain crackers with a little bit of peanut butter
- a handful of cashews and a pear
- a bunch of baby carrots with hummus for dipping
- low-fat yogurt

Equally, if not more important, have a tall, icy-cold glass of water, which will help to take the edge off your hunger, too.

Naomi Campbell told people.com that she sips some mint or lemon tea to fend off cravings.

Skinny Tip

If you are in a rush, you can snack and sip as you are getting ready to go. Either way, make sure snacking happens and you will enjoy the food at your party—and the party itself—without sabotaging your Skinny goals. **SR**

SKINNY RULE

72

Choose Your Drinks Wisely

Next time you're out at a party or a bar, notice what the Skinny girls drink: For the most part, it's wine, light beer, champagne or vodka and soda water. Why? These options have fewer calories than almost any other alcoholic beverage. A glass of wine or vodka and soda water has about 120 calories and champagne and light beer have even fewer—only about 80 calories (or less). Compare this to a traditional martini, which has about 160 calories, or a fancy chocolate martini, which could pile on 430 calories or more!

For a better idea of how many calories you're sipping, check out this handy list, adapted from www.webmd.com, on the following page, which lists drinks in order from heaviest in calories to lightest.

Drink	Serving Size	Calories
Long Island Iced Tea	8 ounces	780
Chocolate Martini	2 ounces each vodka, chocolate liqueur, cream, ½ ounce crème de cacao, chocolate syrup	438
White Russian	2 ounces vodka, 1½ ounces coffee liqueur, 1½ ounces cream	425
Hot Chocolate with Peppermint Schnapps	8 ounces	380
Piña Colada	6 ounces	378
Eggnog with Rum	8 ounces	370
Mai Tai	1½ ounces rum, ½ ounce creme de almond, ½ ounce triple sec, sour mix, pineapple juice	350
Coffee Liqueur	3 ounces	348
Godiva Chocolate Liqueur	3 ounces	310
Margarita	8 ounces	280
Mojito	8 ounces	214
Cosmopolitan	4 ounces	200
Gin and Tonic	7 ounces	200
Vodka and Tonic	8 ounces	200
Screwdriver	8 ounces	190
Beer	12 ounces	150–198

continued

Drink	Serving Size	Calories
Rum and Coke	8 ounces	185
Traditional Martini	2½ ounces	160
Green Apple Martini	1 ounce each vodka, sour apple, apple juice	148
Light Beer	12 ounces	95–136
Port Wine	3 ounces	128
Champagne	5 ounces	106–120
Red or White Wine	5 ounces	120
Bloody Mary	5 ounces	118
Wine Spritzer	5 ounces	100
Rum and Diet Coke	8 ounces	100
Mike's Hard Lemonade	11 ounces	98
Ultralight Beer	12 ounces	64–95
Mimosa	4 ounces	75
Alcohol-Free Wine	5 ounces	20–30

Another Skinny tactic is to mix it up: Between each alcoholic drink, have a glass of water or club soda. Having a drink of water between each alcohol-containing beverage will help to keep you hydrated and your alcohol intake in check.

Or you can use a Skinny splurge tactic and indulge in a cocktail like a lychee martini—but the key is to stop at one. Wondering what a lychee is? A lychee is a tropical Chinese fruit from the soapberry family. Next time you are in the mood for a cocktail, splurge with this Skinny lychee martini recipe:

Skinny Splurge Lychee Martini

Serves 2

Ingredients

⅛ cup Splenda®

¼ cup water

1 cup drained canned lychees (15 to 20, from a 16- to 20-ounce can)

1 ½ tablespoons lemon juice

6 ounces (¾ cup) vodka

1 ounce Peach Schnapps

1 ounce white cranberry juice

Directions

Prepare a heatproof bowl set in a large bowl of ice and cold water. Heat sugar and water in a 1-quart saucepan over high heat, stirring until sugar is dissolved, then pour into the heatproof bowl. Let stand, stirring occasionally, until syrup is cold, about three minutes. Blend lychees with sugar syrup and lemon juice in a blender until smooth, then strain through a fine-mesh sieve into a bowl, discarding solids. Fill cocktail shaker halfway with ice cubes and add lychee purée, vodka, peach schnapps and white cranberry juice. Shake and strain into martini glasses.

Nutrition Facts (per serving)

320 calories, 0 grams fat, 0 grams saturated fat, 0 grams trans fat, 0 mg sodium, 26 grams carbohydrates, 1 gram fiber, 23 grams sugar, 1 gram protein

Recipe adapted from www.epicurious.com.

So if you are going to splurge on a higher-calorie drink, do so in Skinny fashion and limit it to just one! And if you are going to have more than one drink, refer to the list on pages 136–137, stick to lower-calorie options and remember to alternate one alcohol-containing beverage with a glass of water. Both these tips will also help you to keep your alcohol consumption in moderation—for women, one drink per day and for men, two drinks per day. And don't forget, when you have a few too many drinks, your "Skinny guard" may come tumbling down and you could wind up eating unwanted, higher-calorie items just because you have had a few too many drinks! Follow this Skinny rule and put these tips and tricks to use next time you are out on the town and it will surely help you to cut down your calorie intake!

Orange Creamsicle Martini (adapted from Lisa Lillien's recipe)

Serves 1

Ingredients

4 ounces diet orange soda at room temperature

1½ ounces vanilla-flavored vodka

1 ounce sugar-free vanilla syrup

1 tablespoon nonfat Cool Whip

Directions

1. Place all ingredients in a tall glass.

2. Mix gently with a spoon until the mixture is smooth. Add about 1 cup ice and stir until mixture is cold. Enjoy!

For an authentic martini experience, feel free to make in a martini shaker—just stir instead of shaking—and pour into a martini glass.

Nutrition Facts (per serving)

100 calories, 0 grams fat, 0 grams saturated fat, 0 grams trans fat, 0 mg cholesterol, 35 mg sodium, 6 grams carbohydrates, 0 grams fiber, less than 1 gram sugar, 0 grams protein

Recipe adapted from www.lifamilies.com. ⑤ℝ

SKINNY
RULE
73

Plan an Active Vacation

Don't get me wrong, I love to relax on vacation, too, but spending a week on the beach sipping frozen martinis is hardly bikini-friendly! Staying active is the Skinny and surefire way to make room for an extra cocktail or dessert while you are away from home. So how can you transform your vacation into an active vacation? If you're into hiking and nature, seek out nearby walking paths, state parks, local parks, national parks or bike paths. Or plan a vacation that has activity built in, whether it's white-water rafting or skiing. Don't want to pack hiking equipment? Spend time walking around shops, touring the sites or walking instead of taking a cab. Rent a volleyball at the beach and start a pickup game to burn calories while soaking up the sun.

A word of caution: Be sure to plan for an active vacation. Let me share with you a funny example. When my husband, Bill, and I were dating, he lived in the eastern part of the state of Washington. We took an active vacation with his family in the Canadian Rockies (which, by the way, are one of the most beautiful sights you'll ever see). Day #1 we hiked seven miles to a chalet where we were going to camp out in a cabin for the night. Then once we arrived at the chalet, which was a very rustic place, we had to go with a guide and take five-gallon containers to get water from the pump area. And dinner was packets of reconstituted, freeze-dried food because you had to bring in the food; this is where planning ahead comes into play. Know all about the accommodations where you are staying; otherwise, you could wind up getting to your chalet and being surprised that no one is cooking dinner for you. Then Day #2 we hiked over the Continental Divide for another nine miles to the hotel where we were staying the next night.

This is where planning ahead also comes into play. I was in college and did not have the extra cash to buy a new pair of hiking boots for the trek, so I borrowed a pair from a friend for the trip, which fit okay but not perfectly. By the end of the 16 miles, my feet had gotten quite blistered. The lesson: Break in your footwear before vacation and splurge on comfortable footwear (which I have done ever since)— it is totally worth it and it makes a huge difference. The morning after all the hiking, my future husband and I took a three-mile run. I was slowing down toward the end of the three miles (due mainly to my blistered feet). Bill tried to encourage me to keep going and I punched him! Since then I have convinced him to run with me only once, and that was just this past year. If I had had comfortable footwear, perhaps that could have been avoided?!

So when you start planning your active vacation, prepare ahead of time. This will help you pack and will give you an opportunity to familiarize yourself with the area and even seek out some expert help, if needed, like a guided hiking tour. Here are some fun things to consider: Are there any lakes, ponds or rivers around where you can rent boats for a day? Does there happen to be a 5K race while you're in town that you could register for? Are there any nature or wilderness centers that offer guided hikes? Are there national landmarks or special sites unique to the area? Are there walking tours of the city? Is there a bike or walking path nearby? Is there a bike rental place close by? Are skiing or other winter sports available (in the right time of year, of course)?

And if a more rugged active vacation isn't right for you, there are still more luxurious ways to stay active while you are away. Is going to a resort more your speed? When you're at a resort, take the walking path instead of a shuttle! Check out the exercise programs offered there, like yoga,

Pilates or aerobics. Many resorts offer fitness rooms. Find out where they are and visit them! And if weather permits, get in the pool! Leisurely swimming for 30 minutes burns approximately 204 calories.[†] Pack a health magazine that provides simple workouts that you can do without any extra equipment. Have fun next time you leave home and enjoy a more active vacation! ⓢⓡ

<table>
<tr><td>SKINNY
RULE
74</td><td># Drink It Up</td></tr>
</table>

W hile you're soaking up the scenery on your next vacation, remind yourself that staying hydrated is essential, too. While it's fairly easy to drink water in your typical daily routine, it can be a challenge on vacation or while traveling. How much is enough? Sticking with the golden rule of eight cups of water per day for a grand total of 64 ounces of fluid is the goal while at home or on the road. Keep in mind that any type of fluid (except alcoholic beverages) counts toward your daily fluid goal—even coffee and tea.

Why is staying hydrated so essential? Fluid is basically the medium in which all things happen in your body. By the time you are thirsty, your body is actually already 1 percent underhydrated. Your best bet is to "stay ahead" of thirst, so to speak, by routinely drinking fluids throughout the day. This rule is especially important if you are in a warm climate or even at a high altitude, as you will require more water than normal.

And while you can have some natural juice or tea to hydrate, it is still best to stick with mostly water—yes, plain

---

† Based on a 150-pound person.

water. While other calorie-free beverages may be tempting stand-ins for water, nothing beats the real thing. Water too boring or bland for you? Jazz it up with lemon slices, cucumber slices or even raspberries. If you are drinking lots of sugar substitute–sweetened drinks, like diet sodas and teas, challenge yourself to replace a sugar substitute–sweetened drink with water.

Here are some tried-and-true tips to increase your water consumption, especially while you are traveling:

BRING A REUSABLE WATER BOTTLE on vacation to carry along with you during your travels. You can refill the bottle when you are on the go and, as an added bonus, you will be helping the environment, too!

START EVERY MEAL with a glass of icy-cold water. This does a couple of important things. First and foremost, it will help keep you hydrated. Perhaps even more important, it will help take the edge off your appetite, which may result in your consuming less calories.

So tip your glass or water bottle back and keep sipping on icy-cold water throughout the day. Cheers to the new, Skinnier you! ⑤⑫

SKINNY
RULE

75

Back Away from the Buffet

Buffets are notorious Skinny saboteurs, but the truth is the buffet's not to blame: You still have a say in what to eat and avoid, how high you pile your plate and whether you head back for seconds or (eek!) thirds. As a general rule, Skinny girls avoid buffets like the caloriefest they are. But if you wind up at a buffet for one reason or another, navigate it with these Skinny strategies to keep the buffet from getting the best of you.

THE MOST IMPORTANT RULE OF THUMB is one trip only! If you make several trips, you're overeating and consuming unnecessary calories. If you must go back for seconds, grab only fruits or vegetables (and not deep-fried ones). This Skinny rule works because if you are truly hungry, then seconds of fruit or vegetables will do the trick. Otherwise, you are most likely just going back purely because you like the way the food tastes and because it is so easily accessible, rather than out of hunger.

EAT THE SKINNY WAY—SLOWLY. Enjoy your company and carefully chew and actually taste the food you are eating. Have you ever noticed that the thinnest people at the table tend to be the last ones done eating? (See Skinny Rule #13.)

Follow this Skinny rule at parties, too. Rather than grazing and hanging around the buffet all night at your next party, grab one plate (the smallest size available) and fill the smaller-size plate with the snacks and food of your choice. Then—and this is key—once your plate is empty, switch your focus from eating to enjoying the company of those you are with. 🅢🅡

SKINNY RULE **76**

Don't Forget to Go Shopping

When you're traveling for work or play, food is a challenge. The Skinny solution is to go grocery shopping, because, let's face it, eating every meal out is a quick way to pile up tons of extra calories during your vacation. Research shows that you are apt to eat 25 percent more calories when dining out as opposed to eating at home. So when you are away from home, here is what to do: Make a meal plan and choose to eat certain meals at a restaurant, like eating lunch at a restaurant every afternoon.

> Lunch portions at restaurants tend to be smaller than dinner portions, so if you must eat out, lunch is a good meal to choose.

Skinny Tip

Then hit the grocery store to pick up breakfast, snacks and dinner foods. This will allow you to enjoy delicious foods when you are out to eat, yet you will be saving calories (and dollars!) the rest of the day by eating your grocery-bought foods. (If your hotel room doesn't have a refrigerator you can request one or choose shelf-stable foods, like dried fruit, applesauce cups, waxed cheese rounds, peanut butter, whole-grain crackers, ready-to-eat soups and water.) Picking up some healthful foods to keep on hand will help keep the scale in check for when you return home.

In addition to planning meals, stock up on staples to keep on hand, such as fresh fruit and veggies, low-fat milk, yogurt, whole-grain cereal, light cheese spread, whole-grain crackers and granola bars. 🆂🆁

SKINNY
RULE
77

Bring It with You

Don't forget that you can always bring food with you. Remember Skinny Rule #18, Eat Like a Kid? This is the same premise. When kids leave home for any length of time, Mom or Dad makes sure to pack a snack and a drink for the trip. By packing yourself a Skinny snack for the road, you'll have the right type of fuel with you no matter where you are.

As you travel, there will be plenty of tempting, quick, less healthy options readily available for you to grab. In the words of Dr. Jamie Laubisch of Johns Hopkins Medical Center, "Be prepared! For example, if you are going to be traveling via an airport, you know that when you show up there, the food is only going to be premade—that's no secret." Dr. Laubisch also notes that airport food is expensive and often travelers choose things that are full of calories, like a muffin, just because it is convenient, instead of the healthy cereal they would have had for breakfast at home.

Skinny Tip

Travel with a tea bag. Buying tea from a coffee shop is really highway robbery. It's soooo expensive, especially considering that you can buy a box of tea bags for only a few dollars. Instead of buying tea, pack your favorite variety on your next trip and get a cup of hot water instead. Most places won't even charge you for it. It's Skinny and smart!

So use these ideas for simple solutions to bring along on your next trip, whether it is around town, across the country or out for the afternoon. If you arrive with your own grab bag of healthy goodies, you will always be ready to go!

What to pack? Take a cue from style and beauty expert Gretta Monahan, who frequently travels between Boston and New York City. Her trick is to "fill my bags with unsalted nuts and high-protein bars as snacks." These are perfect snacking options, and easy to carry.

Some other simple and tasty travel snack ideas: a handful of pretzels, trail mix (see the recipe below), banana, apple, cheese stick, protein or granola bars and unsalted nuts. You can even pick up some sophisticated, adult-type reusable snack containers or really be like a kid and use ones with cartoon characters on them!

Here is a great Skinny snack that you can make and keep on hand. Pack this trail mix in small baggies so you can just grab one on your way out of the door:

Skinny Trail Mix

Yield: 12 servings

Ingredients

1 cup whole-grain cereal (like Cheerios)

½ cup raisins

½ cup dried cranberries

¼ cup almonds (dry roasted)

¼ cup walnuts (dry roasted)

¼ cup dark chocolate chips

¼ cup sunflower seeds (shelled)

Directions

1. Combine ingredients.

2. Split into 12 quarter-cup servings. Pack in little containers or plastic baggies for a quick grab 'n' go snack.

Nutrition Facts (per serving)

110 calories, 5 grams fat, 1 gram saturated fat, 0 grams trans fat, 0 mg cholesterol, 0 mg sodium, 15 grams carbohydrates, 2 grams fiber, 11 grams sugar, 2 grams protein

Another essential item to bring along is a reusable water bottle. It's a Skinny and green strategy. Keeping well-hydrated is a definite Skinny must! 🅢

Choose These Top Seven Lightest Party Foods

When you are at a party, there are definitely foods to gravitate toward and foods to steer clear of or, at the very least, eat just a small amount of. The best part is that if you are asked to bring something to a party, you can choose something from the list below and you will have a Skinny snack that can be your "go to" goody during the party.

VEGGIE PLATTER: Load up your plate with chopped veggies and skimp on or skip the dip (unless it is hummus). The veggies will provide a satisfying crunch and help fill your belly, too. Plus, the variety of colors adds an antioxidant boost.

FRUIT PLATTER: Fruit is a great option to snack on at a party and certainly among one of the lightest party options. If there is a chocolate or other dipping option, downplay the dip and up the amount of fruit you consume.

SHRIMP COCKTAIL: Just as shrimp is a perfect appetizer option for ordering at a restaurant, it is a great option for parties as well. Choose the shelled variety of shrimp, so they take a little longer to eat, too!

HUMMUS: This tasty dip is made from ground chickpeas blended with extra virgin olive oil, spices and tahini (sesame seed paste). It is a light party food option and, unlike other dips, it provides fiber and protein, both which help to fill you up. And the fat that comes from hummus is mostly healthy, belly-slimming fat. Instead of chips, which will be higher in calories, dip veggies into the hummus.

BRUSCHETTA: Although there are many varieties of bruschetta out there, the traditional blend includes a mixture of chopped tomatoes, spices and extra virgin olive oil, usually served with toasted slices of baguette. This is a tasty, Skinny and delicious party option to enjoy. Just play up the bruschetta and downplay the bread. You can make your own or look for store-bought varieties, too. Enjoy this traditional recipe:

Skinny Bruschetta

Yield: 4 servings

Ingredients

2 cups diced tomatoes (with juice)

4 basil leaves, chopped

2 tablespoons extra virgin olive oil

2 cloves minced garlic

½ cup olives, chopped

Directions

1. Combine all the ingredients.

2. Serve over slices of grilled whole-wheat bread or baguette.

Nutrition Facts (per serving)*

100 calories, 8 grams fat, 1 gram saturated fat, 0 grams trans fat, 0 mg cholesterol, 310 mg sodium, 7 grams carbohydrates, 2 grams fiber, 4 grams sugar, 1 gram protein

*Nutrition data does not include bread or baguette.

SALSA: While salsa has had a "healthy halo" for quite some time, the Skinny word of advice is to dip veggies in the salsa, instead of chips, because one small handful (about 1 ounce) of chips is considered a portion size and will provide about 110 calories and 7 or so grams of fat. So stick to veggies, which are much lower in calories and virtually fat free.

POPCORN: This is my personal favorite party food and it is often on the "menu" when we have guests over. The Skinniest way to prepare it is air-popped and plain. Although, as my husband would tell you, when we have company I do put a little (key words: *a little*) salt and butter on it! The reason why this is a perfect Skinny party food is that 3 cups of popcorn is considered a serving, so your portion lasts a heck of a lot longer than just a handful of chips would. Not to mention, popping your own popcorn works out to cost only about 13 cents per serving, making it an economical choice, too.

Stick with these party foods as a Skinny solution at your next party! 🆂🅿

SKINNY RULE 79

Lighten Up Party Heavyweights

Chances are if I had to ask you what party foods come with a hefty calorie price tag, you could start rattling off quite a few of them. Perhaps they are even some of your favorite foods. The good news is that you can still enjoy your party favorites and splurge every so often (see Skinny Rule #16, Splurge Every Day)—just do so the Skinny way.

It is possible to lighten up some of your favorite party foods—check out these secrets to Skinny-sizing chicken fingers and nachos.

CHICKEN FINGERS: This recipe will result in crunchy and tasty chicken fingers that are so yummy you or your guests won't even miss the deep-fried version. The secret ingredient is the panko bread crumbs—they give the chicken fingers a crispy coating that will taste like they were deep-fried but without all the calories that come along with deep-fried chicken fingers.

Skinny Chicken Fingers

Serves 6

Ingredients

1 pound boneless, skinless chicken tenders

1 cup panko bread crumbs

4 egg whites (whip with a fork)

nonstick olive oil cooking spray

Directions

1. Preheat oven to 350 degrees Fahrenheit.

2. Place whipped egg whites in a dish and the bread crumbs in a separate dish.

3. Spray a skillet with the nonstick cooking spray and warm over medium heat.

4. Dip the chicken fingers into the egg mixture and then into the bread crumbs.

5. Place in the skillet and cook about 4 minutes on each side. Transfer to a baking sheet and bake for about 10–15 minutes or until the chicken is cooked thoroughly.

6. Serve with a barbecue dipping sauce.

Nutrition Facts (per serving)

130 calories, 1 gram fat, 0 grams saturated fat, 0 grams trans fat, 45 mg cholesterol, 100 mg sodium, 7 grams carbohydrates, 0 grams fiber, 0 grams sugar, 21 grams protein

NACHOS: A wonderful party food but the traditional version is loaded with calories and fat. The secret is to make your own, Skinnier version of nachos with this simple recipe.

Skinny Nacho Bowls

Serves 8

Ingredients

1 can refried (low-fat) black beans

1 large chicken breast (4 ounces), cut into bite-size cubes

1 medium red onion, chopped

canola oil

cayenne pepper

10" soft whole-wheat tortilla shells

nonstick olive oil cooking spray

2 plum tomatoes, diced

½ cup grated cheddar cheese, 2%

1 scallion, sliced

¼ cup salsa

¼ cup light sour cream

Directions

1. Preheat the oven to 350 degrees Fahrenheit.

2. Sauté chicken and onion in a small amount of oil (or use nonstick olive oil cooking spray instead) until chicken is browned.

3. Add the black beans to the pan (you may need to add a small amount of water if the beans look dry). Season with cayenne pepper to taste.

4. Place a whole-wheat tortilla in a small, round baking dish and lightly press it in. Bake for about 5 minutes or until golden brown. Remove and place on a serving plate.

5. Fill the freshly baked tortilla "bowl" with the black bean mixture.

6. Top with grated cheese, diced tomato, scallions, salsa and sour cream.

Nutrition Facts (per serving)

140 calories, 4 grams fat, 2 grams saturated fat, 0 grams trans fat, 20 mg cholesterol, 350 mg sodium, 16 grams carbohydrates, 3 grams fiber, 3 grams sugar, 9 grams protein

These are two surefire ways to cut down on the calorie price tag of favorite party foods. There are several other simple swaps you can make to lighten up your next party. Check out the next Skinny rule, Plan a Skinny Party, for more tips and tricks, and revisit Try These Simple Skinny Substitutions (Skinny Rule #58) for more inspiration on easy swaps to lighten things up. 🆂🆁

SKINNY
RULE
80

Plan a Skinny Party

There are secrets to planning a Skinnier party without your guests or you even feeling as if you are missing out on anything at all!

One Skinny strategy is to downplay the focus on food and focus on the reason for getting together to begin with—a movie, the big game, a board game, a card game, catching up with old friends. This shift in focus will help keep the emphasis away from food and more on spending time together—which is more fun than focusing on food anyway!

Another Skinny strategy is to place lighter party fare throughout the room or house; this encourages guests to snack on healthier foods, like veggie trays with salsa for dipping or fruit platters loaded with freshly cut fruit. Put away the mini bowls of candies and nuts. One small handful of nuts, like almonds, constitutes a serving, with a whopping 170 calories (1 ounce). While healthy in moderation, it is very difficult to limit portion size when you have them out in a dish. M&Ms have about 140 calories per small handful (1 ounce)! Not putting out these little extra dishes of foods will help save your and your guests' waistlines. If you must place little dishes around the house, consider some lighter options like Skinny Trail Mix (see Skinny Rule #77, Bring It with You) or even opt for dried fruit, like raisins or dried cranberries, which only have about 80 calories per small handful (1 ounce).

Lastly, follow the 90/10 Skinny strategy: Serve your party guests 90 percent healthier and lighter options and 10 percent more indulgent options. Marcy Blum, a world-renowned event planner and entertaining expert shares her Skinny party rules, which are light, tasty and very clever. Use these ideas to plan your next party with a Skinny flair!

TASTY SOUPS: Blum serves puréed, unthickened, uncreamy veggie soups that are filling and very popular, served chilled or hot, depending on the season, either in a demitasse cup as an hors d'oeuvre or as an appetizer.

JAZZ UP VEGGIE CRUDITÉS: Instead of plain raw vegetables, which can be unsatisfying, Blum recommends blanching vegetables that have been pickled or marinated lightly. Make sure that they are properly drained so that they're not messy, but they still have some flavor.

MAKE YOUR GUESTS WORK A LITTLE: Instead of bowls of shelled nuts, serve nuts in the shell with a nutcracker nearby. This will make it far more difficult to scarf down a pound of them before dinner.

FOR A LIGHT APPETIZER: Include an assortment of whole-wheat summer rolls, which Blum calls "a light and pretty hors d'oeuvre."

AVOID SERVING (OR EATING) CHEESES before dinner: Although tasty, cheese comes with a hefty calorie price tag for a very tiny serving size. Since cheeses are so filling, Blum suggests serving them after the main course with a salad in small portions.

PASTA: Pasta can be a lovely, healthy and filling main course. Use whole-grain pastas and a large ratio of vegetables to pasta. Serve with sauces that are made with a reduction of vegetable stock with a bit of olive oil as a base rather than cream or butter.

Serve your meals in Skinny style. For a buffet, make sure that you have a variety of veggie-based dishes as well as complex carbohydrates and small portions of protein. Arrange the buffet so that the plates are next to the vegetables to begin with. This way, you and your guests will fill up your plate first with veggies and then move onto the heavier foods, like whole-wheat pasta and protein. If you are not into buffet style, family-style service is very much in vogue at the moment, and Blum notes, "Contrary to what you might think, people are less likely to load their plates up in this scenario than if the host places a large portion on each guest's plate."

Blum concludes by offering wine and champagne. As an added touch, choose wines that go with what you are serving. This way people are less likely to ask for sugary mixed drinks.

Now if all this talk has you wondering what to serve for your next party, here is a Skinny hors d'oeuvre plan that is tasty, light and healthy:

BRUSCHETTA served with grilled whole-wheat bread or baguettes for dipping.

FRUIT PLATTER piled with watermelon cubes, cantaloupe and grapes.

POPCORN placed in big bowls throughout your party area, with small serving bowls for guests to scoop popcorn into.

OLIVE PLATTER that includes various types of olives, such as kalmata and black olives, and garlic-stuffed green olives. Be adventurous by trying a new type of olive. Make sure you choose pitted olives to make it easier for your guests to enjoy them.

PIZZA made on whole-wheat crust, cut into bite-size pieces with plain cheese, topped with veggies or black olives.

Stick to smaller-size "appetizer" plates, which will help your guests and you keep your portions in check. The menu above won't leave your guests feeling as if they are missing out on anything; rather, they will enjoy delicious flavors and fill up on Skinnier, healthier options. 🄢

SKINNY RULE 81	Be Better, Not Perfect

In 2007, Tyra Banks launched a "So What!" campaign to encourage women to embrace their bodies, promote positive body images and show that even supermodels can be super-real. In 2006 Americans spent a shocking $12 billion on plastic surgery. As Banks explained to *Good Morning America,* "I have cellulite on the back of my butt. Now I'm starting to get it on my stomach and I don't like it. But I don't stay up at night obsessing about it." As Banks demonstrates, living a Skinny life isn't about being perfect. Those images you see in the magazines are color-corrected and photoshopped to make them *look* perfect. The truth is there's no such thing as "perfect."

So rather than strive for perfection, aim to make better choices. That's the advice of Robyn Priebe, RD, CD, the director of nutrition and program coordinator at Green Mountain at Fox Run, a women's retreat for healthy living without dieting, who recommends that women, "be better, not perfect." What does she mean by that? Make it your goal to improve on your personal "norm," rather than striving to be perfect or comparing your eating habits to others'. Everyone is different and what works for one person won't necessarily work for the next.

Priebe shares an example: Let's say you typically eat four huge slices of deep-dish, meat lover's pizza with extra cheese in one sitting. A practical solution would be to slowly change your way of eating so that you ultimately eat two pieces of thin-crust, plain pizza with a side salad loaded with veggies. The end result is a *huge* change from your personal norm, but you'd set yourself up for failure if you tried to be "perfect" from the start. A Skinny solution would be to slowly cut back until you eventually reached your goal.

Priebe also recommends that you ask yourself, Is this a better choice than what I normally make? If the answer is yes, then you are shifting the delicate calorie balance equation in favor of becoming a Skinnier version of you.

Ultimately, what I'm saying is to cut yourself some slack. Let's face it: Overeating on one occasion is not what causes someone to gain 100, 50, 20 or even 5 pounds. Rather, it is a combination of lifestyle choices and food decisions that result in unwanted pounds. So if you wind up overeating, don't fall into the spiral of shame. Remember, being Skinny isn't just about how you look or what size pants you wear; it is about living a healthier, happier and more fulfilling life! What you need to do is shake it off, and make a better choice next time. 🏵

SKINNY
RULE
82

Plan a Healthy Getaway

Health magazine took a look around the United States to locate the top 10 healthiest beach and lake vacation destinations. Here are their top three locations:

1. **TYBEE ISLAND, GEORGIA:** Exercise is a way of life on the island.

2. **CORONADO, CALIFORNIA:** The judges named this West Coast town "a little slice of heaven." There are tons of ways to get in exercise in Coronado, and trans fats are banned in all restaurants.

3. **MONTEREY, CALIFORNIA:** This won the hearts of the judges, in part, because it is a national marine sanctuary. Some

of the area hotels offer a fitness concierge, while others provide fresh fruit and water in the lobby.

For the rest of the top 10 list, check out www.health.com.

Now, maybe your budget is tight or traveling isn't your thing. The solution can be a staycation, where you take some time off work and have your own version of a vacation without leaving your home. The good news is that there are plenty of ways you can have a healthy vacation without even leaving your home. As Meredith Haberfeld, a New York–based life and career coach told www.health.com, one of the first things you have to do is create a vacation plan and stick to it. She even suggests posting the vacation schedule on your refrigerator. This will help you to feel more like you have escaped from the rituals of your typical everyday routine. It actually can give you an opportunity to enjoy your surroundings by visiting local parks, museums, galleries and other local venues. Taking some time to discover and simply enjoy what is around you can get you feeling connected with your surroundings. If you need help figuring out what is around you, try a free resource— www.discoveramerica.com. ⑱

SKINNY RULE

83

Understand Coffee Shop 101

The menu at coffee shops has exploded, and the calorie content of their drinks has, too! A 16-ounce cup of black coffee has only five calories and zero grams of fat, while the same size blended latte type of drink has about 430 calories and 14 grams of fat.

So what's a Skinny girl to do? Research your favorite coffee drink before you head to the coffee shop to find out its exact calorie price tag. If your favorite coffee joint has a website, that is a great place to find this information. Or talk with the barista to find out how the drink is made. Then before you place your order, you can let her know what you are trying to accomplish: Sugar-free? Nondairy? Low calorie? In many cases, she can steer you in the right direction or customize an existing drink to meet your desired outcomes. The great part now is that most coffee shops are willing to customize their offerings to meet your preferences, so speak up! After all, you're likely paying $3.50 or more for the drink, so make sure you're getting what you want.

Here are some quick ways to shave calories next time you stop to pick up a cup of joe: Skip the whipped! Having whipped cream on top of your drink can add about 120 calories. Ask for your drink to be prepared with nonfat milk; this can save you extra calories as well. Many coffee shops use whole milk or 2 percent milk as the standard milk in their latte drinks. And for the Skinniest of options, choose black coffee or plain tea.

For more information about how many calories are in your favorite coffee shop drinks, check out www.starbucks.com. Keep in mind, however, that calorie counts may vary from shop to shop, depending on their recipe. 🆂🅿

Six

Skinny Eating Out

**SKINNY
RULE
84**

Customize Your Order

There is a Skinny rule to eating out. It starts with how you place an order: The key is to customize. Ordering at face value will get you into trouble almost every time. Start living by this Skinny rule and rarely order something without customizing it to your liking.

Let me give you a prime example. Arby's has a group of offerings on its menu called "Market Fresh," which sounds pretty Skinny. Yet the Market Fresh Roast Turkey Ranch and Bacon Sandwich has cheddar cheese, creamy ranch spread, honey-wheat bread, leaf lettuce, pepper bacon, red onions, roasted turkey and sliced tomatoes. Check out the table below, which lists the calorie price tag that comes with each of the items on the sandwich.

Ingredient	Calories	Fat
Cheddar, slice natural	84	6
Creamy Ranch Spread	166	16
Honey-Wheat Bread	63	7
Leaf Lettuce	3	0
Pepper Bacon	76	6
Red Onions	2	0
Roasted Turkey	117	2
Tomato, sliced	8	0

The creamy ranch spread weighs in at 166 calories and 16 grams of fat. So a first step is, no matter what, start by ordering that sauce on the side. Next, order your sandwich sans cheese, which eliminates another 84 calories and 6 grams of fat. These two changes will save you a total of about 250 calories! Add extra tomato slices for taste and this will only add an extra 8 calories to your sandwich.

If you don't know what comes on the menu item, ask. This will give you a better indication of how you need to customize your order.

Once you have an idea of what the menu item includes, make a quick spreadsheet in your head. Which items have a high-calorie price tag? Which are you willing to do without? With the sandwich example above, maybe you will opt to skip the bacon and instead have cheese on your sandwich. Either way, by skipping some of the high-calorie items, you can Skinny-size your order without sacrificing taste!

Always keep these secret Skinny ordering tips in mind when eating out:

SKIP THE FRIES and instead ask for a side of plain vegetables or a salad. This simple swap can knock off approximately 500 calories. While your meal may still be a high-calorie treat, this will keep it from being a total gut-buster.

CAN'T LIVE WITHOUT THE FRIES? Order a side of fries and a salad (remember Skinny Rule #3, Skip the Sauce, and skip the salad dressing and ketchup).

ORDER THE SMALLEST CUT OF STEAK available on the menu and order it "dry." Steaks taste extra delicious when you eat out because most restaurants top steak with butter, adding an extra 100 calories of pure, unnecessary fat. By ordering your steak dry, you avoid those extra calories.

ASK FOR SAUCES ON THE SIDE: This includes sour cream, butter, dressings, mayonnaise and the like. Then you can be in control of how much of the sauce you add.

Using these tips and tricks will help you to eat out with a lower-calorie price tag while still enjoying your favorite foods. 🅢🅡

Save $$ and Your Waistline

People tend to eat 30 to 50 percent more at restaurants than they do at home, thanks to oversized portions. This rule is all about ordering the Skinny way.

One strategy is to order smaller portions, like appetizers, side dishes, half portions or lunch-size entrées. Most restaurants offer these types of options on their menus and a growing number offer value meals that feature popular menu items at a reduced price and size. Some places even offer mini-dessert options! In general, this is a Skinny strategy to eating out without blowing your calories for the day.

Yet when it comes to selecting appetizers you do still need to proceed with caution. Maybe you were thinking, Yum! A registered dietitian just gave me the green light to order my favorite loaded French fries next time I go out to eat. Of course, there are definitely appetizer selections that I would advise staying away from because they still pack a heavy calorie punch. Avoid fried foods or anything that's loaded with cheese or other fattening additives. At some restaurants, you can even do advance research to find out how many calories are in each menu item.

Here are some of the Skinniest appetizer solutions:

SHRIMP COCKTAIL: In just 3 ounces of shrimp there are only about 80 calories and 1 gram of fat.

QUESADILLA: Sometimes quesadillas can be deadly, but if you order them right, they can be a Skinny choice. Your best bet is to ask for yours to be made with extra veggies, like onions or tomatoes, and skip the sour cream. Opt for salsa just for dipping.

SOUP: Look for noncream-based soups for your lowest-calorie option. Chicken noodle or vegetable soup, for instance, only have about 120 calories per cup.

PIZZA: Not the whole pizza, of course! But share a pizza with your table as a great appetizer. Keep it on the light side by choosing toppings like broccoli, tomatoes or roasted red peppers. And ask for your pizza to be made with less cheese to cut down on the calorie count. Pair it with a side salad and you are good to go.

FRESH BERRIES: If the restaurant has fresh berries on the dessert menu, start your meal with an order of the berries as a sweet, low-calorie treat.

SPRING ROLLS: At Asian-style restaurants, opt for sushi, steamed shrimp, vegetable spring rolls or steamed vegetable dumplings as a great way to start your meal without overdoing it on calories. 🆂🆁

SKINNY
RULE
86

Say That You're Allergic

While food allergies aren't anything to joke about—and can be quite serious in some instances—saying that you're allergic can be one of the best ways to customize your order.

For example, restaurants are notorious for adding butter to foods. Many sit-down restaurants toast your sandwich roll—after giving it a coat of butter first! Most often, cooked vegetables at restaurants are prepared with butter or oil and, in many cases, lots of it. One tablespoon of butter has about

100 calories, 11½ grams of total fat and 7 grams of saturated fat. So your serving of vegetables jumped from about 25 calories and mostly fat free to having as many calories and more fat than a handful of potato chips. Many restaurants coat steaks with butter before they head out to the table to enhance the flavor, but that certainly comes with a heavy calorie price tag.

If you tell your server that you are lactose-intolerant and you need your vegetables and other foods prepared without butter, the restaurant will comply. Ask for your salad without dressing because you're allergic to the ingredients in most dressings. Or mention that you have an allergy to mayonnaise. This will let the server know that it's essential that no butter, dressing or mayo winds up on your plate. 🅢🅡

SKINNY RULE 87
Look for These Skinny Words

How food is prepared has a lot to do with the final calorie price tag of your meal. Because while a whole onion only has about 35 calories, once Outback gets its hands on an onion and turns it into a Bloomin' Onion, it gets transformed into an appetizer that has 1,552 calories! So navigating your way to the Skinniest entrées and menu items has more to do with how it is prepared than anything else. To determine the best meals to order, here are some key Skinny words to look for:

STEAMED: Steaming is a method of cooking whereby food is placed in a steamer basket or rack and cooked over boiling water. No oil or butter is used in the preparation of the food and it is a great way to retain a food's flavor, shape and texture without losing many nutrients.

SAUTÉED: In this cooking method, food is cooked quickly in a small amount of oil in a skillet over direct heat. Note the words *small amount of oil*. This is key because it cooks the food with less added fat than other methods of preparation.

BAKED: Foods are cooked in an oven by surrounding them with dry heat. This is a great way to order chicken and fish, since dry heat means that it is typically not covered in butter or oils to cook. Make sure you mention that you want no butter or oil added. Ask for butter to be served on the side only or use Skinny Rule #86 and tell your server that you are allergic to butter.

GRILLED: When foods are grilled, they are cooked on a grill over hot coals or another heat source. The word *barbecue* is often used synonymously with *grill*. Look for steak, shrimp, vegetables, fish, chicken and pork prepared this way.

BROILED: Broiled foods are cooked directly under the heat source. Many foods can be prepared this way, adding great flavor and very little fat. This is a terrific way to order fish, in particular.

Foods tend to be prepared differently from restaurant to restaurant, so if you're in doubt, ask your server about how the food is prepared. This can help you decipher if the menu item is something that is loaded with extra calories or if it is a Skinny option. 🆂🆁

SKINNY
RULE
88

Avoid These Un-Skinny Words

J ust as there are words to look for on a menu, there are words to avoid, too. I'm sure you can think of some of these words off the top of your head, but there are many words that are code for high-calorie foods. Here are some of the heavier hitters to avoid when you are ordering, or customize them by following other Skinny rules to make them lighter:

CREAMY: When it comes to soups and sauces, *cream-based* means costly in the calorie balance equation. *Bisque* is code for creamy; one cup of lobster bisque may have about 260 calories and 18 grams of fat!

DEEP-FRIED: It is hardly surprising to learn that deep-fried foods are higher in calories and fat than their baked or broiled counterparts. In the case of potato chips, innocent potatoes go from being a virtually fat-free food to 1 ounce (a small handful) having 110 calories and 10 or so grams of fat.

SMOTHERED WITH CHEESE: While cheese provides calcium, protein and other essential nutrients, when a food is smothered with cheese, it is also smothered with calories and fat. One ounce of cheese has about 120 calories and 9 grams of fat, so the smothering of your food with cheese could add an extra 360 calories and 27 grams of fat (or more!) to the dish in a hurry. If you must order something with the words *smothered with cheese* in the description, ask for a light amount of cheese to be used.

TENDER: You will see this word pop up often under the meat selections on a menu. What makes meat tender? Fat. The leanest cut of steak to opt for is filet mignon.

LOADED: While this could be a good thing if the restaurant were referring to food piled high with vegetables, the word *loaded* often comes with a huge calorie price tag! For example, a loaded baked potato soup has about 290 calories and 18 grams of fat per cup. And over half the fat is coming from artery- and heart-clogging saturated fat.

Next time you are reading a menu, look at it a little differently and watch out for some of these key words that are likely to deliver a whopping amount of calories in your bowl or on your plate. 🆂🅿

SKINNY
RULE
89

Pick Your Poison

This rule is all about making choices, trade-offs or, as I like to say, picking your poison. As you know, I believe in splurging (see Skinny Rule #16), but you should weigh your options to avoid overdoing it.

What do I mean by picking your poison? Here's an example: Recently my husband and I attended a state fair, which was crawling with fried food and calorie-loaded options around every corner. So we decided to splurge wisely. The "poison" we picked was sharing a few different fried options from one vendor and a barbecue pulled pork sandwich without French fries from another vendor (we'd already had our share of fried food "poison").

Practice this rule the next time you're at a restaurant or fast food joint. Eying the French fries and a bacon cheeseburger? Pick your poison and choose one high-calorie item with a side of plain steamed vegetables or a leafy green salad. Have it prepared without butter and keep the sauce on the side. If you are out to eat with a group of people who like to enjoy a multicourse meal, from appetizers to dessert, pace yourself and pick your poison. Maybe you have a sweet tooth? If that is the case, skip the appetizer and save some calories for dessert. If you love appetizers, carefully choose your meal starter and then, when it is time for dessert, choose an herbal tea or coffee in place of a high-calorie, gooey dessert.

This counts for drinks, too! That margarita and fried meal are double trouble—choose one or the other.

So do the Skinny thing and pick your poison—you'll be surprised to see just how easy it can be to make these trade-offs. ⑤ℝ

SKINNY RULE
90

Share with a Friend

Put this rule into practice when you go out to eat and it will definitely help you save calories. The trouble with eating out is that it's difficult to avoid overeating with the monstrous serving portions most restaurants serve. By splitting an entrée, you ensure that you're eating a reasonable portion—and you'll save money while you're at it.

If you are not into sharing, ask your server to box up half your meal before it ever arrives to your table. This will enable you to be less likely to overeat once your food arrives. Then take the other half of your meal home and have it for dinner or lunch the next day. This is a particularly good Skinny strategy for dessert. Definitely share your dessert with someone else, and even consider sharing with the whole table! Here's an insider secret for you: Registered dietitians almost always order dessert when eating out together. We just make sure to share it.

Start sharing, too, and your waistline will thank you! ⑤🅡

SKINNY RULE
91

Just Ask

You know you need to customize your order, so here are additional Skinny strategies to do so.

First of all, ask if you don't know. Do you know what béarnaise sauce is? It is a very rich sauce that is made of clarified butter and egg yolks and typically seasoned with tarragon, shallots, chervil (an herb related to parsley) and simmered in vinegar. If you don't know how a food is prepared or what the sauce is made of, just ask. Your server will describe the menu item and its preparation so you can make a more informed decision.

Another key reason to just ask is because foods are prepared differently in restaurants than you would prepare them at home, and the preparation will even vary from restaurant to restaurant. Once you ask, you can make more informed decisions and alter your order to save calories. Remember, too, to just ask if smaller portions are available. This is an especially good strategy for dinner. As another added benefit, you may save a little cash, too; the smaller portions will often come with a reduced price tag. ⑤

Seven

Skinny Fashion

<table>
<tr><td>SKINNY
RULE
92</td><td># Choose the Right Colors, Prints and Patterns</td></tr>
</table>

Why does every woman own a little black dress? Because black is among the most slimming colors. Wearing figure-flattering colors is a Skinny must. If you are not into black, that's okay; the deep-colored hues of dark blue, purple and brown create the same kind of slimming illusion.

This goes for denim, too. Say goodbye to faded and acid-washed denim and choose jeans with dark washes for an instantly slimming look.

Steer clear of colors like white and khaki that visually add on the pounds. Khakis are especially unhelpful if you are trying to slim down wide hips.

Beyond these general rules, there are some basic Skinny tips on how you can use color to your advantage. The most important thing to keep in mind is that wherever you are placing the emphasis, bring colors; you are most definitely drawing attention to that area. Want to minimize your bottom half? Go with dark jeans or black pants and wear a pop of color on top to draw the eye upward. Top-heavy? Go with a white or khaki skirt and a dark top to balance things out. Trying to look overall slimmer? Avoid bright-colored clothing altogether; instead choose a brightly colored handbag or jewelry instead.

Perhaps one of the best ways to use color to your advantage is to dress in monochromatic colors from top to bottom. Using one color from top to bottom will create a visual illusion that lengthens the body—it's a perfect solution for petite frames, in particular. Pairing a light- or bright-colored top with dark pants will visually cut the body in half, making a short person appear even shorter!

What about stripes and patterns? The Skinny rule is to never, ever choose horizontal stripes unless you're looking to add 10 pounds to your frame. Vertical stripes can actually be your best friend, as they can hide figure flaws and help you to appear taller and thinner. Some great options to try: a deep-purple blouse with vertical stripes and a black skirt, or a chocolate-brown top with chocolate-brown pinstriped pants.

And always avoid wearing the same print on top and bottom to avoid looking like a giant flower print. Instead, pair your flowered top with a pair of black pants and your flowered capris with a coordinating solid top. And remember that prints and patterns draw attention, so wear them strategically.

The trick is to make colors, prints and patterns work for you and not against you. §

SKINNY RULE 93 Know Your Body

There's one thing Skinny girls know really well and that's their body. Whether top-heavy or hippy, petite or tall, there are strategies to maximize assets and minimize trouble spots for any body type.

George Simonton, acclaimed fashion designer and professor at the Fashion Institute of Technology, says it best: "You must, bottom line, take a cold hard look at yourself." He explains that most women do not look at themselves from head to toe before they leave the house in the morning and this is where the problem starts. Women really need to look at the whole package, not just their face or the upper part of their body.

Simonton shares some interesting statistics: The average American woman is 5-foot-4½ inches tall, wears a size 12 top and a size 14 bottom. What works for models may not work for you—and what works for you may not work for your friend. You need to know your body shape and work with it, rather than working against it when it comes to fashion.

What are your best features? Your so-called "problem areas"? Once you know your body type, play up your best features, regardless of your size. Simonton suggests:

To show off wonderful legs: Play them up with beautiful shoes.

To camouflage not so wonderful legs: DO NOT wear skirts.

To show off a beautiful face: Focus on the neckline and play up the face with accessories.

To camouflage ample arms: Keep sleeves light and airy, like "butterflies."

To camouflage a big tush: Look for jackets with open side seams to downplay the bum.

To elongate your neck: Use beautiful long chains and necklaces.

To elongate your face: Sweep hair up over the ear and opt for chandelier earrings.

Judie Schwartz and Evelinda Urman are columnists and bestselling authors, who present seminars on all aspects of professional image. Schwartz and Urman share Simonton's philosophy and recommend embracing your body type first and foremost: "We have never met a woman who didn't think her body could be improved in some way. Think of clothing as a figure optical illusion that accentuates the positive and camouflages the negative." Their best advice is to dress for the body you have now. Here are a few of their insider tips:

If you have no waist: Wear belts.

If you have curvy hips: Balance your body's shape with fitted tops that float over your hips and definitely wear darker-colored bottoms.

If you have a full chest: Elongate your torso with unadorned, open-neck tops and dresses, and avoid high necklines.

Additionally they suggest forging a close relationship with a tailor. And remember: Inexpensive, well-fitting clothes look better than expensive ill-fitting ones. Don't buy something simply because it is in style or looks good on someone else, unless it is right for you.

Lastly, when losing weight, go through your closet and ditch the clothes that don't fit anymore. This way you won't slip back into the bigger size that you left behind. Say goodbye to it, donate the clothes and use these tips to pick out new clothes to flatter the Skinny new you! 🆂🅿

| SKINNY RULE **94** | # Finishing Touches Go a Long Way |

There are little fashion finishing touches that will help you look your best and slimmest at any size.

Rule number one: Improve your posture and stand up tall! For every inch you slouch, you look like you weigh five pounds more. On the flip side, standing up tall with good posture will make you look five pounds slimmer instantly. As Elizabeth G. Griswold, AAFA, a group fitness instructor, explains, the added bonus to standing and sitting up straight is that "good posture will visually melt inches from your midsection." To improve your posture, she suggests adding yoga and/or Pilates to your workout regimen two to three days a week for 30 to 45 minutes. You'll gain the muscle strength and muscle memory for your body to hold itself taller and straighter, thereby looking longer and leaner. Plus, the physical and mental benefits will make you feel and look great.

Rule number two: If you want to add height to your figure, opt for a three-inch heel and always try on before you buy—if you can't walk gracefully in the heel, you're just going to look awkward and the extra height won't be worth it!

Rule number three: Finish your outfit with a pointy-toed shoe—it will help to elongate the body, making you appear taller and Skinnier. 🅢🅡

SKINNY RULE

95

Wear the Right Size

Skinny girls always wear clothes that fit properly and are cut best for their body. It may be tempting to squeeze into a smaller-size pair of jeans to feel thinner, but you'll actually wind up bulging out of them and looking *heavier*. The same goes for wearing loose, baggy clothes: They *really* add on the pounds. The way to look your slimmest, no matter what your size, is to wear tailored clothes that fit your body.

However, finding clothes that fit is quite difficult today because of vanity sizing. As a result, it may feel as though you are trying to put a square peg into a round hole. George Simonton, a tenured professor of fashion design at New York's Fashion Institute of Technology, notes, "There are designers that put a size 4 on a size 8 garment, which may make it hard to know which size is the right size." Here is what Skinny girls do: Pay less attention to the size on the label and pay even more attention to how the garment fits you. Use these tips as your "Does this really fit me well?" checklist:

NO PINCHING: If any part of an article of clothing pinches or causes part of your body to "spill" over, opt for a larger size or forget the garment altogether. Maybe it just isn't right for you.

NO PULLING: When choosing shirts, make sure there isn't too much pulling in the bust area. If there are buttons on the top, watch for any pulling. When it comes to pants make sure that the zipper and/or button lie flat and do not pull.

NO PUCKER: With jackets, pay close attention to how the shoulders lie. If there is any puckering, choose a larger size or a style that better fits your shoulders.

Choosing the right size holds true when it comes to accessories, too. Skinny people know that balanced accessories can actually make you look thinner. For example, if you're a larger person and you choose a thin belt or a tiny purse, you are actually drawing attention to your size. Instead, try a medium-sized purse, a wide belt or a large necklace. Along the same lines, petite girls should avoid oversized accessories.

The bottom line is to make your clothing and accessories work for you. Pay less attention to the size label and focus on whether it really fits. Keep the three Ps in mind: no *pinching, pulling* or *puckering*. ⓢⓡ

SKINNY
RULE
96

Define You

Fashion expert Sharon Harver says it best: "If Jennifer Lopez hid her round butt and big boobs, we would never have heard of her! Thank Miss J.Lo for making it OK to be built like a brick house and be proud of it. Flaunt those womanly curves."

To make your mark, Harver explains that you must accept the body you have and make the most of what you've got to feel great about yourself. She emphasizes that baggy clothes do no one any good: "By all means, dress like you give a darn when you leave the house!"

Harver's rule of thumb is that clothing should act like a second layer (not too big or too small) to your body that emphasizes what you want to highlight and camouflages what you want to play down.

Then, she says, you must "Go out and have some fun. Laugh. Frolic. Have a swell time. Think about how thrilling life could be the next day. Then, go shopping. If you are in less of a funk, your clothing choices will be less tedious and more alive."

Remember, you are in charge of what you buy. And you don't have to fall victim to every whim of fashion—especially if tiny belts won't work on your long torso or chunky necklaces will make you look that much more petite! Hate wearing high heels? Then don't! You can be just as fashionable in flats. Part of making your mark is learning who you are, what looks best on you and what feels most natural.

Perhaps most important, as Harver explains, "No matter how fabulous your wardrobe is, it's still just clothing. Gorgeous clothes and a dreary outlook still make a dull person." Project an air of self-confidence and poise and what you're wearing will suddenly look better. 🆂🆁

SKINNY RULE 97 | Make Over Your Look

Life is busy, and it's easy to get so caught up in the day-to-day to-do list that you forget to think about yourself. But fashion changes—from colors to cuts—and clothes wear out. There's nothing like a makeover to lift you up and bring out your Skinny side.

For the how-to on redefining your look, I checked with the Style Matters gals, Judie Schwartz and Evelinda

Urman. Evelinda states, "We are all about high style at low prices and redefining your look can be easily done on a budget." She explains that the first thing you need to do is make an honest assessment of your appearance. Ask yourself: Am I still wearing the same clothes I wore five years ago? Have I updated my hairstyle in the last two years? Have I bought a new lipstick or eyeliner in the last few years? If you answered yes to the first question and no to the last two, here are some simple, inexpensive Style Matters' tips for updating your look:

MAKE OVER YOUR MAKEUP: Makeup trends change every season, so the Style Matters gals suggest opting for a more natural timeless look to get the most out of your makeup budget. They even recommend considering a professional makeup consultation or going to a cosmetics counter for a free makeover. If you feel guilty about taking advantage of the free service, buy a lipstick. Select a lipstick closest to your lip color for a natural, everyday look.

> Improve your smile and look years younger by whitening your teeth. A good smile is always flattering—no matter how far along you are on your Skinny goals.
>
> **Skinny Tip**

JUDIE AND EVELINDA: Don't fret about your figure flaws—the right clothing can help you accentuate the positive and camouflage the negative. Most important, dress for the body you have now and develop a close relationship with a tailor.

BRUSH UP YOUR HAIR! When was the last time you changed stylists? If it has been a while, then it is time to pick someone with a new perspective on your face shape, hairstyle and color. A couple of Skinny rules of thumb: Avoid center parts because they emphasize asymmetrical facial features and choose styles that have layers to add movement and thickness to your hair.

The bottom line is that style matters! Judie and Evelinda say, "Trust us. When you update your look, you not only look better, you feel better. And that's what fashion is really all about." 🆂🆁

Find *Your* Skinny Jeans

Big butt? Flat butt? Long legs? Short legs? You name it—there are certain jeans that are right or wrong for you. Even though you may be tempted to purchase a new pair of denim because they are a certain designer brand or look really cute on a friend, it's more important to choose clothes for your body than to follow the latest fad. How do you find your personal Skinny jeans? Here are some tried-and-true tips:

Flat butt: If you have a flat butt, flare cuts will work for you, especially if you want to minimize your thighs. Fitnessmagazine.com recommends mid- and low-rise styles to make sure your bottom doesn't sag.

Boyish figure: High-waist styles will be perfect for you to add some curves and ankle-cut jeans work well, too.

Tall and curvy: Wide-leg jean styles will be your best choice.

Full thighs: Trouser-style jeans will minimize thighs, thanks to the full legs.

Full hips and thighs: Go for a fitted cut and choose a pair of jeans with a longer hem. Alternatively, mega-flare jeans will help balance out hips and thighs.

Short legs: You can give short legs a longer look with a straight-leg jean. Paired with a pointed-toe shoe, it will help to trick the eye into seeing one long line.

Long legs: Stick to low- to mid-rise jeans so you are not elongating your legs further. Be sure to find jeans that come in longer cuts to accommodate your longer legs.

Petite: Skinny jeans work well for you to add curves and show off your figure. Or look for ankle-cut jeans; as an added bonus, you can show off your shoes.

Plus sizes: Choose straight or flared jeans for a flattering look; the best bet are types that fall across your natural waist.

Big tush: Angled pockets can work wonders by creating a slimming illusion on the bum.

Going for a relaxed look? Opt for a boyfriend cut, which works for all body types.

According to www.marieclaire.com, the winning jean cut that works universally to flatter almost any figure is the boot cut. And don't forget: Jeans look best when hemmed to the shoe height you normally wear. The longer the line, the taller and thinner you'll look.

Happy jeans shopping, and here's to feeling great in your next pair of denim! 🆂🆁

SKINNY RULE 99

Make Your Accessories Work for You

Every Skinny girl has an arsenal of smart accessories to pull her look together. The trick is to use accessories to accentuate the positive rather than drawing attention to the negative, explains Ellen Goldstein, chairperson of the Accessory Design Department at the Fashion Institute of Technology. Here is what you need to know:

Handbags

Goldstein recommends choosing a bag to "fit your stature." If you are petite, use a shorter strap as opposed to a long strap; if you are tall or heavier, you can choose a larger bag with a shorter strap. While she suggests that almost everyone can carry large or oversized bags, Goldstein's word of caution is to make sure you do not overstuff them, as this will affect your posture. And be sure not to carry too many bags.

Belts

Goldstein explains that belts come and go in fashion and how and what is in style varies as well. Yet there are general Skinny rules of thumb to stick to: "If you are tall or slim, you can wear thin and tightly cinched belts." If you are heavier, she suggests that you be conscious of how the belt fits and go for more of a draped look. Stay away from belts that cinch tightly.

Shoes

The Skinny rule of thumb is to alternate your shoes between flats and heels. As Goldstein explains, when you wear flats, your Achilles tendon stretches out, so rather than just wearing flats all the time, swap your flats for heels from time to time to lessen the stretching of your Achilles tendon. Good news, tall girls: You don't have to shy away from heels! But avoid heavy and chunky-heeled shoes if you are heavier. And if you are going to wear flip-flops or open-toed shoes, you *must* give your toes a pedicure.

Jewelry

"Jewelry should be worn proportionately to your body size," explains Goldstein. Large beads are really in style right now, but huge beads look ridiculous on a petite person. Instead, if you are petite, go for a scaled-down version of the look for the same effect, but in a more flattering way. This goes for watches and bracelets, too.

Accessorize with Color

Goldstein loves color—"color is wonderful"—and she recommends using color to detract from flaws and accentuate your best features. For example, choose a scarf or handbag with color. Think about where you are placing the color. If you are wearing an all-black dress and add a hot-pink belt, it will certainly draw attention to your midsection, which is great for girls who want to draw attention to their midsection, but not for girls who want to minimize it. ⓢⓡ

SKINNY
RULE
100

Frame Your Face

Believe it or not, there is such a thing as Skinny hair! From updos to length, here are your hair dos and don'ts:

Elongate the face: Fashion guru George Simonton notes that elongating the face helps you look slimmer. One of his tips is to wear the hair up over the ear and put on a pair of chandelier earrings to create a slimming look. New York City salon owner Mark Garrison told *Fitness* magazine that "sleek, midlength strands" will help you look 10 pounds thinner because it lengthens your face.

Additional slimming hairstyles and looks to go for include collarbone length–cut hair; opt for bangs that are slightly angled, choose choppy ends with few layers and go for a straight texture. For a straight look, Garrison suggests using a straightening balm and use the balm starting at your roots all the way to your ends. When you are blow-drying your hair, do so in sections. While drying your hair to maximize the smoothing effect, try using a paddle brush or a round, metal-based brush—either option will help to smooth hair much as a flatiron does. Before you finish drying your hair, if your dryer has a cool setting, switch to that to help maintain a smooth look as it will seal the cuticle of the hair, which will help to keep it looking smooth. To finish the slimmed-down Skinny look, use a flatiron and end with a bit of antifrizz serum or an all-over-shine spray.

When in doubt, talk with your stylist about what look is right for you to help play up your features and frame your face! ⓢⓡ

Eight

Conclusion

SKINNY RULE 101

Customize Your Skinny Life

Now that you have read 100 Skinny rules, it is time to put the rules into action in your life, and make your own personalized Skinny action plan. Perhaps you are going to start at the beginning with Rule #1, Believe You Can Be Skinny. Or maybe you are going to jump in and start at Rule #52, Don't Forget the Magic Meal. That is the best part about this book: You can choose your own Skinny adventure. Most important, pick and choose the rules that work for you, as every reader will start reading this book at a different point in her life.

As you put the Skinny rules to work for you, here are a few reminders:

IT TAKES TIME TO FORM A NEW HABIT and how long it takes will depend on what type of habit you are trying to form. So don't be too hard on yourself and keep on trying! If you have a "bad" meal or snack, no worries. Just get started back on your Skinny plan with the next meal or snack.

SKINNY is defined by the lifestyle you lead, not by the number on the scale or what size clothes you wear.

THE RULES YOU NEED TO FOCUS ON will change from time to time as your life changes, so keep this book in a convenient spot. That way, you can pull it out to focus and redefine your Skinny plan as you need to.

It may sound too simplistic that all you need to do is follow these rules to live a Skinny life, yet that is truly how simple it can be. And know that you can create a healthier version of yourself! **SR**

Appendix A

Skinny Experts

Mark Blanchard, yoga expert and creator of True Power Yoga DVD, www.truepoweryoga.com

Marcy Blum, world-renowned event planner and entertaining expert

Gretta Cole, fashion and beauty expert, www.grettastyle.com

Keri Gans, RD, nutrition expert and American Dietetic Association spokesperson

Michael George, celebrity personal trainer

Ellen Goldstein, chairperson of the Accessory Design Department at the Fashion Institute of Technology

Elizabeth G. Griswold, AAFA, group fitness instructor

David Grotto, RD, LDN, nutrition expert and author of *101 Optimal Foods*

Rich and Helen Guzman, co-owners of L.A. R.O.X and trainers for Hilary Swank

Sharon Harver, fashion guru, www.focusonstyle.com

Dr. David Katz, director and co-founder of the Yale Prevention Research Center, www.davidkatzmd.com

Eric Khron, chef and registered dietitian

Dr. Jamie Laubisch, Johns Hopkins Medical Center

Robin Miller, host of the Food Network's *Quick Fix Meals* and author of *Robin Rescues Dinner*

Paulette Mitchell, author of 14 cookbooks, including *The Complete 15-Minute Gourmet: Creative Cuisine Fast and Fresh*

William Morgan, MS, PT, physical therapist

The Nutrition Twins®, Tammy Lakatos Shames, RD, LD, CDN, CPT, and Lyssie Lakatos, RD, LD, CDN, CPT, co-authors of *The Secret to Skinny: How Salt Makes You Fat and the 4-Week Plan to Drop a Size and Get Healthier with Simple Low-Sodium Swaps*

Robyn Priebe, RD, CD, director of nutrition and program coordinator at Green Mountain at Fox Run Spa

Linda Quinn, MS, RD, CDN, registered dietitian and spokesperson for New York Apple Association, www.nyapplecountry.com

Cynthia Sass, MPH, MA, RD, CSSD, New York City–based registered dietitian and bestselling coauthor of the *Flat Belly Diet!*

George Simonton, acclaimed fashion designer and a tenured professor at the Fashion Institute of Technology

The Style Matters gals, Judie Schwartz and Evelinda Urman, www.stylematters.us; stylematters@comcast.net

Liz Vaccariello, editor-in-chief of *Prevention* and coauthor of the *Flat Belly Diet!*, www.flatbellydiet.com

Robyn Webb, MS, cookbook author, food editor of *Diabetes Forecast* magazine and coauthor of the recently published *Dr. Barnard's Get Healthy, Go Vegan Cookbook: 125 Delicious Recipes to Jump Start Your Weight Loss and Feel Great*

Lisa Young, PhD, RD, author of *The Portion Teller Plan,* www.portionteller.com

Elisa Zied, MS, RD, CDN, spokesperson for the American Dietetic Association and author of *Nutrition at Your Fingertips* and *Feed Your Family Right!*

Appendix B

Skinny Tools

Throughout this book, I refer to many Skinny tools, including books and websites. Here is a complete listing of those tools and more to help you along your way to becoming a healthier you.

America on the Move: www.americaonthemove.org

American Dietetic Association: www.eatright.org

Calorie Count: www.caloriecount.about.com

CalorieKing: www.calorieking.com; search this site's "Food Database" to see the nutrition facts for food items and restaurant meals.

Caloriesperhour.com: Click on "Calories Burned Calculator" to quickly calculate, based on your weight, how many calories you burn by doing a variety of activities, from accordion playing to yoga.

Center for Science in the Public Interest: www.cspinet.org

CookingLight magazine: www.cookinglight.com

Discover America: www.discoveramerica.com

Dr. Andrew Weil: www.drweil.com

EatingWell magazine: www.eatingwell.com

Epicurious: www.epicurious.com

Fitness magazine: www.fitnessmagazine.com

Food Network: www.healthyeats.com

Food Network: www.foodnetwork.com

Health magazine: www.health.com

Joke of the Day: www.joke-of-the-day.com

Lé Scoop (Bagel Scooper):
www.jambsupply.com/lescoop.html

LIFamilies: www.lifamilies.com

Map My Ride: www.mapmyride.com

Map My Run: www.mapmyrun.com

marie claire magazine: www.marieclaire.com

Mayo Clinic: www.mayoclinic.com; a great tool for calculating your target heart rate(s).

Mayo Clinic: www.mayoclinic.org

Men'sHealth magazine: www.menshealth.com

MyPyramid (Food Guide Pyramid): www.mypyramid.gov

Online nutrition database: www.nutritiondata.com

National Institutes of Health, Body Mass Index Chart: www.nhlbi.nih.gov

National Sleep Foundation: www.nationalsleepfoundation.org

Natural Resources Defense Council: www.nrdc.org

NowLoss: www.nowloss.com

People magazine: www.people.com

Prevention magazine: www.prevention.com

Rachael Ray: www.rachaelray.com

Running information: www.runnersworld.com

Self magazine: www.self.com

Shape magazine: www.shape.com

Starbucks: www.starbucks.com; a Skinny favorite to see how many calories are in your favorite coffee shop drinks. You can also see how the calories change when you customize your drink, like ordering without whipped cream and changing the serving size.

True Power Yoga DVDs: www.truepoweryoga.com

WebMD: www.webmd.com

Women'sHealth magazine: www.womenshealthmag.com

Appendix C

Skinny References

Introduction
Fitness magazine, Alison Sweeney, host of *The Biggest Loser,*
http://www.fitnessmagazine.com
(Accessed September 11, 2009).

Skinny Rule #2
National Sleep Foundation, "How Much Sleep
Do We Really Need?" http://www.sleepfoundation.org
(Accessed July 23, 2009).

C. A. Crispim, et al., "The Influence of Sleep and
Sleep Loss Upon Food Intake and Metabolism,"
Nutrition Research Reviews 20, no. 2 (2007): 195–212.

Skinny Rule #4
Heidi Klum, "Here's How 24 Celebrities Lost Weight
After Having Their Babies..." http://www.nowloss.com
(Accessed July 16, 2009).

Skinny Rule #6
University of Texas Health Science Center at San Antonio,
"New Analysis Suggests 'Diet Soda Paradox'—Less Sugar,
More Weight," http://www.uthscsa.edu
(Accessed July 23, 2009).

Skinny Rule #10
James K. Binkley, "Calorie and Gram Differences between
Meals at Fast Food and Table Service Restaurants," *Applied
Economic Perspectives and Policy* 30, issue 4 (2008): 750–763.

Ruby Tuesday, "Nutritional Menu Guide,"
http://www.rubytuesday.com
(Accessed October 13, 2010).

Burger King, http://www.bk.com
(Accessed October 13, 2010).

Skinny Rule #11
SELFNutritionData, "Nutrition Facts: Yogurt, Plain,
Low Fat, 12 Grams Protein Per 8 Ounce,"
http://nutritiondata.self.com
(Accessed July 28, 2009).

SELFNutritionData, "Nutrition Facts: Salad Dressing, Mayonnaise, Imitation, Soybean," http://nutritiondata.self.com (Accessed July 28, 2009).

Skinny Rule #15
NutriBase 8 Professional Edition, v.8.3.8, 1986 to 2010 by Cybersoft, Pheonix, A2.

Skinny Rule #16
People magazine, "Easy Celeb Diet Tips," http://www.people.com (Accessed August 26, 2009).

Skinny Rule #17
Vanderbilt University Medical Center, "No Joke: Study Finds Laughing Can Burn Calories," http://www.mc.vanderbilt.edu (Accessed September 12, 2009).

"Angel's Food vs. Devil's Food," http://www.joke-of-the-day.com (Accessed September 12, 2009).

Skinny Rule #19
B. Wansink, et al., "Ice Cream Illusions: Bowls, Spoons, and Self-Served Portion Sizes," *American Journal of Preventive Medicine* 31 (2006): 240–243.

Skinny Rule #21
American Yoga Association, http://www.americanyogaassociation.org (Accessed April 26, 2010).

Skinny Rule #23
CNN, "The Celebrity Trainer Approach to a More Perfect Body," http://www.cnn.com (Accessed September 14, 2009).

Phillippa Lally, et al., "How Are Habits Formed: Modelling Habit Formation in the Real World," *European Journal of Social Psychology* (2009).

Skinny Rule #25
Dovico Software, "Tips & Whitepapers, Time Management Facts and Figures," http://www.dovico.com (Accessed August 3, 2009).

Skinny Rule #26

Fitness magazine, "Kristi Yamaguchi's Pilates Workout," http://www.fitnessmagazine.com
(Accessed September 12, 2009).

People magazine, "What Is Brooke Shields' Secret to Being Fit?" http://www.people.com
(Accessed August 26, 2009).

Fitness magazine, "The Britney Spears Workout: How She Got Her Body Back," http://www.fitnessmagazine.com
(Accessed September 12, 2009).

Fitness magazine, "Kristi Yamaguchi's New Pilates Body," http://www.fitnessmagazine.com
(Accessed September 12, 2009).

Skinny Rule #27

Fitness magazine, "Hilary Swank's Arm and Shoulder Exercises," http://www.fitnessmagazine.com
(Accessed September 14, 2009).

Skinny Rule #31

Fitness magazine, "Get a Hot Body," http://www.fitnessmagazine.com
(Accessed September 15, 2009).

Gunnar Borg, *Borg's Perceived Exertion and Pain Scales,* Champaign, IL., Human Kinetics, 1998.

Skinny Rule #33

Training Calendar, http://www.mapmyride.com
(Accessed September 14, 2009).

Training Calendar, http://www.mapmyrun.com
(Accessed September 14, 2009).

Skinny Rule #34

Mayo Clinic, "Target Heart Rate Calculator," http://www.mayoclinic.com
(Accessed September 14, 2009).

Training Calendar, http://www.mapmyride.com
(Accessed September 14, 2009).

Training Calendar, http://www.mapmyrun.com
(Accessed September 14, 2009).

William D. McArdle, et al., *Exercise Physiology: Energy, Nutrition, and Human Performance,* 7th Edition, Lippincott, Williams & Wilkins, 2009.

Skinny Rule #35
People magazine, "Ashley Tisdale: Gym 'Felt like Torture,'"
http://www.people.com
(Accessed August 2, 2009).

Skinny Rule #36
Mayo Clinic, "Whole Grains: Hearty Options for a
Healthy Diet," http://www.mayoclinic.com
(Accessed October 1, 2009).

"The Story," http://www.arnoldpalmertee.com
(Accessed October 1, 2009).

Skinny Rule #37
BeHollywoodFit.com, "Marisa Miller Avoids Processed
Foods," http://www.behollywoodfit.com
(Accessed October 13, 2010).

Michael Pollan, *In Defense of Food: An Eater's Manifesto,*
Penguin Books, 2008.

Skinny Rule #38
Dr. Andrew Weil, "Choosing Foods by Color,"
http://www.drweil.com
(Accessed October 1, 2009).

Skinny Rule #40
Prevention magazine, "Sassy Water," http://www.prevention.com
(Accessed September 14, 2009).

Newsweek, "Six Facts about Belly Fat,"
http://www.newsweek.com
(Accessed September 14, 2009).

Heather I. Katcher, et al., "The Effects of a Whole-
Grain-Enriched Hypocaloric Diet on Cardiovascular
Disease Risk Factors in Men and Women with Metabolic
Syndrome," *American Journal of Clinical Nutrition,* 87
(2008): 79–90.

Skinny Rule #41
Yunshen Ma, et al., "Association between Eating Patterns
and Obesity in a Free-living US Adult Population,"
American Journal of Epidemiology, no. 158 (2003): 85–92.

USA Today, "An Apple a Day Keeps the Calories at Bay,"
http://www.usatoday.com
(Accessed October 13, 2010).

Skinny Rule #44
http://caloriecount.about.com
(Accessed on August 20, 2009).

Skinny Rule #45
Center for Science in the Public Interest, "Chemical Cuisine, Learn About Food Additives," http://www.cspinet.org
(Accessed April 26, 2010).

U.S. Department of Health and Human Services, Butylated Hydroxyanisole (BHA), http://www.ntp.niehs.nih.gov
(Accessed April 26, 2010).

Skinny Rule #46
Time magazine, "Getting Real About the High Price of Cheap Food," http://www.time.com
(Accessed September 16, 2009).

Skinny Rule #47
New York Times, "For Your Health, Froot Loops," http://www.nytimes.com
(Accessed September 16, 2009).

NuVal, http://www.nuval.com
(Accessed October 13, 2010).

Skinny Rule #48
Self magazine, "Snacks of the Stars," http://www.self.com
(Accessed September 12, 2009).

Skinny Rule #51
Lisa Young, *The Portion Teller Plan: The No-Diet Reality Guide to Eating, Cheating, and Losing Weight Permanently.* New York: Morgan Road Books, a division of Doubleday Broadway, Random House, May 2005.

Skinny Rule #52
National Weight Control Registry, http://www.nwcr.ws
(Accessed October 13, 2010).

Skinny Rule #53
Dr. David Katz, "Plant Foods in the American Diet? As We Sow..." *Medscape Journal of Medicine* 11, no. 1 (2009): 25. http://www.pubmedcentral.nih.gov
(Accessed September 16, 2009).

Natural Resources Defense Council, "Eat Local: Does Your Food Travel More Than You?" http://www.nrdc.org (Accessed September 16, 2009).

Skinny Rule #54
Progressive Power Yoga, "About Yoga," http://www.progressivepoweryoga.com (Accessed October 1, 2009).

Skinny Rule #55
Yunshen Ma, et al., "Association between Eating Patterns and Obesity in a Free-living US Adult Population."

James K. Binkley, "Calorie and Gram Differences between Meals at Fast Food and Table Service Restaurants."

Skinny Rule #56
Brian Wansink, *Mindless Eating: Why We Eat More Than We Think*. New York: Bantam Dell, 2006.

Skinny Rule #61
United States Department of Agriculture, http://www.fsis.usda.gov (Accessed August 7, 2009).

Skinny Rule #66
Definition of Sous-Chef, http://www.merriam-webster.com (Accessed October 13, 2010).

Skinny Rule #71
People magazine, "How Pregnant Stars Stay Fit," http://www.people.com (Accessed October 13, 2010).

Skinny Rule #72
People magazine, "Easy Celeb Diet Tips," http://www.people.com (Accessed August 26, 2009).

WebMD, "Low-Calorie Cocktails," http://www.webmd.com (Accessed September 2, 2009).

"Skinny Splurge Lychee Martini" from http://www.epicurious.com (Accessed October 13, 2010).

LIFamilies, "Skinny Martinis: Figure Friendly Cocktails," http://www.lifamilies.com (Accessed October 13, 2010).

Skinny Rule #73

Activity Calculator, http://www.caloriesperhour.com
(Accessed October 8, 2009).

Skinny Rule #80

Nutrition Facts for M&Ms, http://nutritiondata.com
(Accessed September 11, 2009).

Nutrition Facts for Almonds, http://nutritiondata.com
(Accessed September 11, 2009).

Nutrition Facts for Raisins, http://nutritiondata.com
(Accessed September 11, 2009).

Skinny Rule #81

Fitness magazine, "Celebrity Workout Secrets: 17 Fitness
Tips," http://www.fitnessmagazine.com
(Accessed September 14, 2009).

Good Morning America, "Tyra Banks Says 'So What!'"
http://abcnews.go.com
(Accessed September 14, 2009).

Skinny Rule #82

Health magazine, "7 Ways to Have a Healthy Vacation
Without Ever Leaving Your Home," http://www.health.com
(Accessed September 28, 2009).

Health magazine, "American's Healthiest Beach and Lake
Getaways," http://www.health.com
(Accessed September 28, 2009).

Skinny Rule #83

Starbucks Beverage Details, http://www.starbucks.com
(Accessed September 3, 2009).

Skinny Rule #84

Food Dictionary, http://www.epicurious.com
(Accessed September 3, 2009).

Arby's Nutrition Facts, http://www.arbys.com
(Accessed September 8, 2009).

Skinny Rule #85

B. J. Rolls, "The Supersizing of America: Portion Size and
the Obesity Epidemic," *Nutrition Today* 38 (2003): 42–53.

"NRA Survey of Chefs Reveals Top Food Trends
Heating Up on Restaurant Menus," http://www.restaurant.org
(Accessed September 8, 2009).

New York Post, "Read Calorie Count and Weep,"
http://www.nypost.com
(Accessed September 3, 2009).

Calorie Count for Shrimp, http://www.nutritiondata.com
(Accessed September 8, 2009).

Calorie Count for Chicken Noodle Soup,
http://www.nutritiondata.com
(Accessed September 3, 2009).

Skinny Rule #87
Outback Steakhouse, Interactive Nutritional Menu Tool,
http://www.outback.com
(Accessed October 13, 2010).

Skinny Rule #88
Souplantation and Sweet Tomatoes' Soups: Loaded
Baked Potato with Bacon, http://www.calorieking.com
(Accessed September 11, 2009).

Zoup!'s Soups, Lobster Bisque, http://www.calorieking.com
(Accessed October 8, 2009).

Skinny Rule #91
Definition of Béarnaise Sauce, http://en.wikipedia.org
(Accessed September 27, 2009).

Skinny Rule #98
Style magazine, "A Jean Come True,"
http://www.stylemagazine.com
(Accessed September 24, 2009).

marieclaire magazine, "Jeans That Fit Your Body—Real
Women in Real Fashion," http://www.marieclaire.com
(Accessed September 24, 2009).

Fitness magazine, "Jean Therapy: The Best Jeans for Every
Body," http://www.fitnessmagazine.com
(Accessed September 24, 2009).

Fitness magazine, "Good Jeans: The Perfect Jeans for Your
Body," http://www.fitnessmagazine.com
(Accessed September 24, 2009).

Skinny Rule #100
Fitness magazine, http://www.fitness-digital.com
(Accessed October 13, 2010).

Index